T0259193

Small Animal Theriogenology

Guest Editors

CATHERINE G. LAMM, DVM, MRCVS
CHELSEA L. MAKLOSKI, DVM, MS

VETERINARY CLINICS OF NORTH AMERICA: SMALL ANIMAL PRACTICE

www.vetsmall.theclinics.com

May 2012 • Volume 42 • Number 3

SAUNDERS an imprint of ELSEVIER, Inc.

W.B. SAUNDERS COMPANY
A Division of Elsevier Inc.

1600 John F. Kennedy Blvd. • Suite 1800 • Philadelphia, PA 19103-2899

http://www.vetsmall.theclinics.com

VETERINARY CLINICS OF NORTH AMERICA: SMALL ANIMAL PRACTICE Volume 42, Number 3
May 2012 ISSN 0195-5616, ISBN-13: 978-1-4557-3957-8

Editor: John Vassallo; j.vassallo@elsevier.com

Veterinary Clinics of North America: Small Animal Practice (ISSN 0195-5616) is published bimonthly (For Post Office use only: volume 42 issue 1 of 6) by Elsevier Inc., 360 Park Avenue South, New York, NY 10010-1710. Months of issue are January, March, May, July, September, and November. Business and Editorial Offices: 1600 John F. Kennedy Blvd., Ste. 1800, Philadelphia, PA 19103-2899. Customer Service Office: 3251 Riverport Lane, Maryland Heights, MO 63043. Periodicals postage paid at New York, NY and additional mailing offices. Subscription prices are $283.00 per year (domestic individuals), $455.00 per year (domestic institutions), $138.00 per year (domestic students/residents), $375.00 per year (Canadian individuals), $559.00 per year (Canadian institutions), $416.00 per year (international individuals), $559.00 per year (international institutions), and $201.00 per year (international and Canadian students/residents). To receive student/resident rate, orders must be accompained by name of affiliated institution, date of term, and the signature of program/residency coordinator on institution letterhead. Orders will be billed at individual rate until proof of status is received. Foreign air speed delivery is included in all *Clinics* subscription prices. All prices are subject to change without notice. **POSTMASTER:** Send address changes to *Veterinary Clinics of North America: Small Animal Practice,* Elsevier Health Sciences Division, Subscription Customer Service, 3251 Riverport Lane, Maryland Heights, MO 63043. Customer Service (orders, claims, online, change of address): Elsevier Periodicals Customer Service, Elsevier Health Sciences Division, Subscription Customer Service, 3251 Riverport Lane, Maryland Heights, MO 63043. Tel: 1-800-654-2452 (U.S. and Canada); 314-447-8871 (outside U.S. andCanada). Fax: 314-447-8029. E-mail: journalscustomerservice-usa@elsevier.com (for print support); journalsonlinesupport-usa@elsevier.com (for online support).

Reprints. For copies of 100 or more of articles in this publication, please contact the Commercial Reprints Department, Elsevier Inc., 360 Park Avenue South, New York, NY 10010-1710. Tel.: 212-633-3812; Fax: 212-462-1935; E-mail: reprints@elsevier.com.

Veterinary Clinics of North America: Small Animal Practice is also published in Japanese by Inter Zoo Publishing Co., Ltd., Aoyama Crystal-Bldg 5F, 3-5-12 Kitaaoyama, Minato-ku, Tokyo 107-0061, Japan.

Veterinary Clinics of North America: Small Animal Practice is covered in *Current Contents/Agriculture, Biology and Environmental Sciences, Science Citation Index, ASCA, MEDLINE/PubMed (Index Medicus), Excerpta Medica,* and *BIOSIS.*

Printed and bound by CPI Group (UK) Ltd, Croydon, CR0 4YY

Transferred to Digital Print 2012

Contributors

GUEST EDITORS

CATHERINE G. LAMM, DVM, MRCVS
Diplomate, American College of Veterinary Pathologists; School of Veterinary Medicine, University of Glasgow, Bearsden, Glasgow, United Kingdom

CHELSEA L. MAKLOSKI, DVM, MS
Diplomate, American College of Theriogenologists; JEH Equine Reproduction Specialists, Whitesboro, Texas

AUTHORS

CANIO BUONAVOGLIA, DVM
Department of Veterinary Public Health, Faculty of Veterinary Medicine of Bari, Bari, Italy

LELAND E. CARMICHAEL, DVM
James A. Baker Institute for Animal Health, Cornell University, Ithaca, New York

BRUCE W. CHRISTENSEN, DVM, MS
Diplomate, American College of Theriogenologists; Assistant Professor, Department of Veterinary Clinical Sciences, Iowa State University, Ames, Iowa

NICOLA DECARO, DVM, PhD
Department of Veterinary Public Health, Faculty of Veterinary Medicine of Bari, Bari, Italy

ROBERT A. FOSTER, BVSc, PhD, MACVSc
Diplomate, American College of Veterinary Pathologists; Professor, Department of Pathobiology, Ontario Veterinary College, University of Guelph, Guelph, Ontario, Canada

ELIZABETH M. GRAHAM, MVB, MVM, PhD, MRCVS
Academic Head of the Infectious Diseases Diagnostic Laboratory, University Veterinary Clinician; School of Veterinary Medicine, College of Medical, Veterinary and Life Sciences, University of Glasgow, Glasgow, United Kingdom

EDUARDO GUTIÉRREZ-BLANCO, DVM, MSc
Associate Professor of Medicine and Clinical Pharmacology, Department of Animal Health and Preventive Medicine, Autonomous University of Yucatan, Yucatan, Mexico

MATILDE JIMÉNEZ-COELLO, DVM, MSc, PhD
Associate Professor of Veterinary Infectious and Parasitic Diseases, Department of Molecular Biology, CIR-Biomedicas "Dr Hideyo Noguchi", Autonomous University of Yucatan, Yucatan, Mexico

CATHERINE G. LAMM, DVM, MRCVS
Diplomate, American College of Veterinary Pathologists; School of Veterinary Medicine, University of Glasgow, Bearsden, Glasgow, United Kingdom

CHERYL LOPATE, MS, DVM
Diplomate, American College of Theriogenologists; Reproductive Revolutions, Aurora; Wilsonville Veterinary Clinic, Wilsonville, Oregon

CHELSEA L. MAKLOSKI, DVM, MS
Diplomate, American College of Theriogenologists; JEH Equine Reproduction Specialists, Whitesboro, Texas

HERRIS S. MAXWELL, DVM
Diplomate, American College of Theriogenologists; Clinical Professor, Department of Clinical Sciences, College of Veterinary Medicine, Auburn University, Auburn, Alabama

BRADLEY L. NJAA, DVM, MVSc
Diplomate, American College of Veterinary Pathologists; Department of Pathobiology, Oklahoma State University, Stillwater, Oklahoma

ANTONIO ORTEGA-PACHECO, DVM, MVSc, PhD
Professor of Animal Reproduction Small and Large Animals, Department of Animal Health and Preventive Medicine, Autonomous University of Yucatan, Yucatan, Mexico

MARGARET V. ROOT KUSTRITZ, DVM, PhD
Diplomate, American College of Theriogenologists; Professor, Vice-chair, Veterinary Clinical Sciences; Assistant Dean of Education, University of Minnesota College of Veterinary Medicine, St Paul, Minnesota

FRANCES O. SMITH, DVM, PhD
Diplomate, American College of Theriogenologists; President, Orthopedic Foundation for Animals, Inc., Columbia, Missouri; Owner, Smith Veterinary Hospital, Burnsville, Minnesota

DAVID J. TAYLOR, MA, PhD, VetMB, MRCVS
Diplomate, European College of Porcine Health Management; Diplomate, European College of Veterinary Public Health; Emeritus Professor of Veterinary Bacteriology and Public Health, University of Glasgow, Glasgow, United Kingdom

ROBYN R. WILBORN, DVM, MS
Diplomate, American College of Theriogenologists; Assistant Professor, Department of Clinical Sciences, College of Veterinary Medicine, Auburn University, Auburn, Alabama

Contents

FORTHCOMING ISSUES

July 2012

Geriatrics
William D. Fortney, DVM,
Guest Editor

September 2012

Minimally Invasive Fracture Repair
Brian Beale, DVM,
Guest Editor

November 2012

Ear Disease
Bradley Njaa, BSc, DVM, MVSc, and
Lynette Cole, DVM, PhD,
Guest Editors

RECENT ISSUES

March 2012

Common Toxicologic Issues in Small Animals
Safdar A. Khan, DVM, MS, PhD, and
Stephen B. Hooser, DVM, PhD,
Guest Editors

January 2012

Hematology
Joanne B. Messick, VMD, PhD,
Guest Editor

November 2011

Companion Animal Medicine: Evolving Infectious, Toxicological, and Parasitic Diseases
Sanjay Kapil, DVM, MS, PhD,
Guest Editor

RELATED INTEREST

Veterinary Clinics of North America: Exotic Animal Practice
May 2012 (Vol. 15, No. 2)
Pediatrics
Kristine Kuchinski, DVM, PhD, *Guest Editor*

Preface

Small Animal Theriogenology

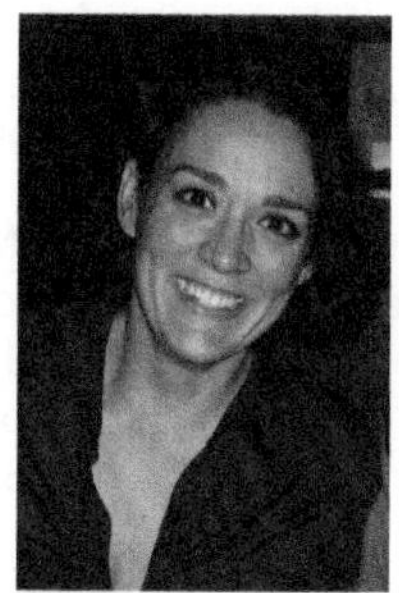

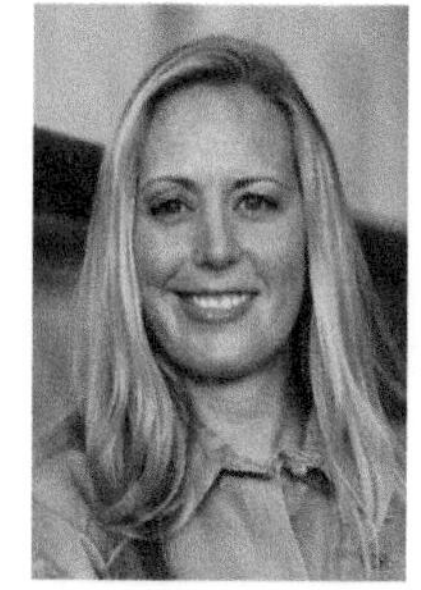

Catherine G. Lamm, DVM, MRCVS Chelsea L. Makloski, DVM, MS
Guest Editors

For this issue of the *Veterinary Clinics of North America: Small Animal Practice*, international leaders in the field of veterinary theriogenology have joined to create a comprehensive, state-of-the-art edition that explores the various aspects of reproductive health and disease in the dog and cat. Theriogenology in dogs and cats has advanced rapidly in the last decade, with the development of new techniques to increase pregnancy rates and promote the full-term birth of a healthy litter.

The articles are organized in a linear fashion, from conception to birth, providing guidance in cases of both traditional and complicated reproductive cases. The emphasis in this issue is on breeding and parturition. However, later articles deal specifically with reproductive disease in the dog and cat and are applicable to both breeding and nonbreeding animals. We hope that this issue will be an excellent addition to your practice library and work as a reference for you in the management of breeding animals and treatment of reproductive diseases.

We thank Elsevier/Saunders for this opportunity and John Vassallo for his assistance in its development and production. The editors would also like to thank the contributing authors for their hard work and creation of an outstanding edition. Dr Cathy Lamm would like to thank Dr Donald Schlafer for nurturing an interest in reproductive pathology and Dr Brad Njaa for never-ending support and encouragement. Dr Chelsea Makloski would like to thank Drs Reed Holyoak and Michelle

Vet Clin Small Anim 42 (2012) ix–x
doi:10.1016/j.cvsm.2012.02.002

LeBlanc for opening the door to the world of theriogenology and Dr Peggy Root-Kustritz for her guidance and support in the area of small animal theriogenology.

Catherine G. Lamm, DVM, MRCVS
School of Veterinary Medicine
University of Glasgow
Bearsden, Glasgow
G61 1QH, UK

Chelsea L. Makloski, DVM, MS
JEH Equine Reproduction Specialists
1030 Roland Road
PO Box 650
Whitesboro, TX 76273, USA

E-mail addresses:
Catherine.Lamm@glasgow.ac.uk (C.G. Lamm)
cmakloski.jehers@yahoo.com (C.L. Makloski)

Managing the Reproductive Cycle in the Bitch

Margaret V. Root Kustritz, DVM, PhD

KEYWORDS

• Bitch • Reproduction • Estrus • Breeding management

This article reviews the normal physiology and endocrinology of the estrous cycle of the bitch and how to use that information to guide decisions about breeding management. This article also explains the mechanism of action of pharmaceuticals and strategies for estrus induction and suppression. There are many excellent review articles published on these topics. The references cited here include some of those review articles, from which readers may locate articles from the primary literature if they wish, and recent publications. Topics that will not be addressed are general methods of contraception and pregnancy termination.

THE CANINE ESTROUS CYCLE

The canine estrous cycle consists of 4 recurring stages (**Table 1**).[1] *Proestrus* is defined as the first outward evidence of fertility in the bitch. *Estrus* is defined by the bitch's behavior; she will allow the male to mount and breed her during this stage. For this reason, many owners call this stage "standing heat." *Diestrus* is defined as the bitch no longer being receptive to mounting and breeding ("going out of heat"). The end of diestrus is defined as a decline in progesterone below that needed to maintain pregnancy (1 to 2 ng/mL [3.1 to 6.2 nmol/L]).[2,3] *Anestrus* is defined as absence of outward signs of fertility and low serum progesterone concentrations.[1]

The *interestrous interval* is defined as the duration from onset of a given proestrus to onset of the subsequent proestrus. Interestrous interval varies between bitches and may vary within bitches, with reported average of 6 to 7 months and reported range of 5 to 12 months.[3] Underlying causes of variation in interestrous interval include breed and environment. German shepherd dogs and rottweilers frequently are described as having interestrous intervals shorter than the average, although one study refutes this in one population of German shepherd dogs.[4,5] Basenjis and Tibetan mastiffs cycle only once yearly, and some populations of wild dogs also may cycle seasonally, with time of estrous activity such that pups are born during clement weather early enough in the season so they are full grown before seasonally inclement weather redevelops.[3,6,7] Domestic

The author has nothing to disclose.

Veterinary Clinical Sciences, University of Minnesota College of Veterinary Medicine, 1365 Gortner Avenue, St Paul, MN 55108, USA
E-mail address: rootk001@umn.edu

Vet Clin Small Anim 42 (2012) 423–437
doi:10.1016/j.cvsm.2012.01.012 **vetsmall.theclinics.com**
0195-5616/12/$ – see front matter

Table 1
Parameters of the canine estrous cycle

Stage (Duration)	Physical Changes	Behavioral Changes	Vaginal Cytology	Primary Endocrine Event(s)
Proestrus (9 d, range 3–21 d)	Vulva swollen and turgid, serosanguinous vulvar discharge	Males interested, bitches will not allow mount or breeding	Gradual increase in percentage cornified cells, decrease in PMNs	Follicular development; rise in serum estrogen concentration
Estrus (9 d, range 3–21 d)	Vulva softens, straw-colored vulvar discharge	Bitch allows mount and breeding	All cells cornified with greater than 50% anuclear, no PMNs	Fall in estrogen with subsequent rise in LH and ovulation, preovulatory rise in progesterone
Diestrus (pregnant bitches 62–64 d, nonpregnant bitches 49–79 d)	Slight mucoid discharge early in diestrus, mammary development possible with true or false pregnancy	None	Abrupt return to noncornified epithelial cells, large number of PMNs early in stage	Progesterone rises and then falls over this stage, falling abruptly at end (pregnant dogs) or more gradually diminishing (non-pregnant dogs). Progesterone production is supported by LH and prolactin secretion.
Anestrus (1–8 mo)	None	None	Noncornified epithelial cells, occasional PMNs	FSH relatively elevated throughout, LH concentrations increase late in stage after estrogen priming

bitches generally are described as nonseasonal in their estrus activity, although one study demonstrated some seasonality dependent on exposure to natural light and temperature.[3,4] Studies disagree as to whether interestrous interval is dependent on whether the bitch became pregnant and whelped.[4,5]

Puberty in bitches is defined as the first overt sign of fertility and therefore usually is defined as the first obvious proestrus. Time of puberty varies with breed, with small breed bitches entering estrus as early as 4 months of age and giant breed bitches as late as 2 years of age. Average range for onset of puberty in bitches is 6 to 14 months of age.[3]

Proestrus

The bitch's owner or handler is the person who usually identifies onset of proestrus, using the physical clues of turgid vulvar swelling and serosanguinous vulvar discharge. The author recommends that owners watch for vulvar discharge as that is a more definable sign than is swelling and so is easier to note consistently from one cycle to the next. This serosanguinous discharge arises from the uterus, by extravasation of red blood cells (RBCs) through endometrial venules.[8] Amount of vulvar discharge varies between bitches and neither an unusually small nor an unusually large amount is associated with subfertility or infertility. Owners call the onset of proestrus "coming into heat," and when an owner says a bitch has "been in heat" for so many days, they are saying it has been that many days since onset of proestrus. Male dogs are interested in urine and vulvar secretions from bitches in heat and may approach and try to investigate her hindquarters or mount her. The bitch will not permit mounting or breeding during proestrus, which lasts an average of 9 days but may last anywhere from 3 to 21 days.[1,3]

Ovarian follicles are undergoing maturation during this stage of the cycle as they transition from secondary, or preovulatory follicles, to tertiary follicles, also called ovulatory or Graafian follicles. Ovulatory follicles are large (>4 mm in diameter) and lined with granulosa cells that produce estrogen.[9] The primary form of estrogen secreted in bitches is estradiol-17β. It is this estrogen that is responsible for the physical changes of proestrus described earlier, and that will stimulate the vaginal epithelium to divide, causing characteristic changes in vaginal cytology that will be described with breeding management. Serum estradiol concentrations peak at values of 50 to 100 pg/mL during this stage of the cycle.[1]

Estrus

Estrus most often is defined by owners by evaluating the behavior of experienced males, many of whom will not show significant interest in a bitch until she is receptive to breeding and near her fertile period, and the behavior of the bitch, who will permit the male to mount and breed her during this stage of the cycle. Classically, the vulva softens as the bitch enters estrus, and the vulvar discharge changes in color from serosanguinous to straw-colored. Owners often call this "the color change" and worry if it does not occur. Some bitches will have vulvar turgidity and serosanguinous discharge throughout estrus, with no apparent effect on fertility. Estrus lasts an average of 9 days, with a possible range of 3 to 21 days.[1,3]

Ovarian follicles in bitches undergo preovulatory luteinization, a process whereby granulosa cells and surrounding theca cells in the follicles change morphologically and start to produce small amounts of progesterone.[2] Coincident with this, there is a decline in serum estrogen concentrations. This triggers release of a large pulse of luteinizing hormone (LH) from the pituitary, which stimulates ovulation 36 to 50 hours later.[1,10] After ovulation, serum progesterone concentrations continue to rise.

Diestrus

All bitches go through a prolonged luteal phase with significant progesterone production whether they were bred or not and whether they conceived and established pregnancy or not. Vulvar discharge wanes as the bitch no longer permits mounting and breeding behavior; in some bitches, a small to moderate amount of mucoid discharge may be passed early in diestrus. Because progesterone concentrations are high during this stage, bitches may show physical changes owners may attribute to pregnancy whether or not the bitch is pregnant. These include mammary development and, in some bitches, rib spring with apparent abdominal enlargement. Elevated progesterone concentrations also are associated with uterine changes appropriate for pregnancy, including endometrial hyperplasia and increased secretory activity of endometrial glands. Diestrus lasts an average of 50 to 80 days.[3] If the end of diestrus is defined by decline in progesterone to <1 to 2 ng/mL, the length of diestrus in pregnant dogs averages 62 to 64 days from ovulation as progesterone falls abruptly at the time of whelping. In nonpregnant dogs, diestrus may be prolonged as there may be a more variable decline in serum progesterone concentrations, such that diestrus may last anywhere from 49 to 79 days from ovulation.[2] It has been shown that corpora lutea (CLs) no longer produce progesterone after 60 to 120 days from ovulation but may be visible on the ovary until the next proestrus.[11]

All progesterone during this stage of the cycle is produced by CLs formed at the ovulation sites on the ovaries. These CLs are maintained spontaneously early in diestrus but are dependent on secretion of LH and prolactin from the pituitary in the latter half of diestrus.[2] Secretion of progesterone from luteal CLs is stimulated by LH and prolactin may play a role by suppressing ovarian responsiveness to follicular development.[10,12] It is not clear what is the driving force in luteal regression in dogs. Prostaglandin release may play a role as may decline in LH and prolactin. Opioids also may be involved, perhaps through association with secretion of luteotrophic LH.[2]

Anestrus

Anestrus has historically been considered a time of reproductive quiescence. It is now better understood that while there are no outward signs of reproductive activity during this stage, there are histologic and endocrine changes occurring that are required for onset of the next proestrus. Involution of the uterus takes 135 days (4.5 months), and this is the minimum length of anestrus considered normal in dogs.[7] Reported ranges for anestrus range from 1 to 8 months.[3] Serum concentrations of follicle stimulating hormone (FSH) remain stable throughout anestrus at anywhere from 50 to 100% of preovulatory concentrations, and while there are FSH receptors present on the ovary, follicular development is suppressed until very late in this stage.[10,13] Serum estrogen concentrations rise slightly in late anestrus. This rise in estrogen primes the hypothalamo-pituitary-ovarian axis, causing increased responsiveness to gonadotropin releasing hormone (GnRH) and subsequent increases in frequency and magnitude of pulses of LH secreted.[10,14] This stimulates follicular growth and the onset of the next proestrus.

BREEDING MANAGEMENT

Several factors unique to bitches make breeding management more challenging than in other species. Because we have limited access to the ovaries physically or visually, we must infer what is happening on the ovaries by diagnostic testing. Bitches ovulate an immature oocyte, which must undergo one more meiotic division before it can be fertilized. For this reason, optimal breeding is offset from ovulation day. Proestrus and estrus are prolonged, with behavioral estrus not well correlated with ovulation. Many of the diagnostic tests used approximate the day of ovulation but only endocrine assays provide the general practitioner with any accuracy in prospectively determining ovulation day. Increasing accuracy is required with increasing sophistication of insemination. With natural breeding or use of fresh semen, spermatozoa may live in the bitch's reproductive tract for up to 1 week, making them available whenever ova have matured and can be fertilized.[3] With chilled semen, life span of spermatozoa decreases to days, and with frozen/thawed semen, to hours, necessitating accurate timing of ovulation and subsequent insemination.

Duration of Estrous Stages/Breeding Management History

The average bitch is in proestrus for 9 days and ovulates about the second day of estrus. For this reason, many people breed bitches on days 9, 11, and 13, counting day 1 as the onset of proestrus and assuming they have an average bitch. There is great variability between bitches and one cannot assume that all bitches bred over this window are being bred near their most fertile time; it is reported that bitches may first show behavioral estrus anywhere from 2 days before to 5 days after the LH peak that causes ovulation and that number of days from proestrus onset to ovulation may vary from 5 to 30.[1,15] Once a bitch has had ovulation date determined, usually by measurement of progesterone as described later, breeders may assume that she will ovulate on about that same day of her cycle repeatedly. This has not been demonstrated to be true.[15] The author prefers to use history to help determine when to see the bitch for breeding management rather than as a predictor of events in this cycle; for example, if a given bitch ovulated very late in her last season, the owner probably does not need to rush in with the bitch on the second day after proestrus onset in this cycle.

Physical Changes

As described previously, vulvar tone and characteristics of the vulvar discharge vary as the bitch progresses from proestrus into estrus. The average bitch shows these changes at the onset of estrus and ovulates about 2 days later.[15] However, there is great variability and, again, one cannot use this parameter alone to accurately determine ovulation day.

Vaginal Cytology

Under the influence of estrogen, vaginal epithelial cells are stimulated to divide. As samples are collected over the estrous cycle, characteristic changes in cell populations are noted (**Table 1**).

The author collects vaginal cytology specimens using a nonsterile, cotton-tipped applicator that is moistened with tap water. The swab is inserted dorsally in the vulvar cleft and passed craniodorsally at a 45° angle, to bypass the ventral clitoral fossa. The swab is passed until it passes the pelvis and can be directed more cranially, is rolled gently against the vaginal wall, and then removed. The swab is rolled several times over a clean glass slide. The slide is allowed to air-dry and then routinely stained. Cells are examined under the ×10 objective.

Four epithelial cell types are identified. Parabasal cells are those lining the basement membranes (**Fig. 1**). They are round with a 1:1 or smaller cytoplasm:nucleus ratio. Intermediate cells lie above parabasal cells (see **Fig. 1**). They also are round with a large, well-defined nucleus and are slightly larger than parabasal cells. These are the noncornified epithelial cell types and are always present in the vagina. As epithelial cell division is stimulated by elevated serum concentrations of estrogen in proestrus, a layer of nonviable cells develops as the vaginal epithelium thickens. Histologically, there will be 5 to 7 layers of parabasal and intermediate cells covered by 4 to 6 layers of keratinized cells.[16] Because the swab collects cells from the lumen, only these keratinized cells will be collected. Superficial cells and anuclear squames are the keratinized or cornified cell types. Superficial cells are misshapen and angular and have a pyknotic nucleus (**Fig. 2**). Anuclear squames are superficial cells with no visible nucleus (see **Fig. 2**).

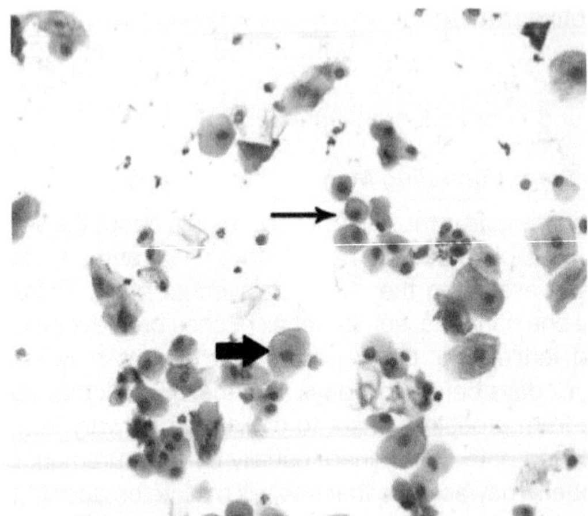

Fig. 1. Early proestrus vaginal cytology from a bitch. Note parabasal epithelial cell (*small arrow*) and intermediate epithelial cell (*large arrow*).

During proestrus, percentage cornified cells increases gradually and the number of polymorphonuclear cells (PMNs) decrease. RBCs may be present throughout. Estrus is defined cytologically as presence of 100% cornified cells types with at least 50% of those being anuclear squames (**Fig. 3**). No PMNs are present and there are variable numbers of RBCs and bacteria. Ovulation occurs on the second day of estrus in the average bitch, but this timing is widely variable and should not be relied upon for prospective timing of ovulation day, since peak in cornification can occur anywhere from 5 days before to 1 day after the LH peak.[3] Six days after ovulation, the cornified cell layers are abruptly sloughed off, such that noncornified epithelial cells are recovered on cytology. Many PMNs are present in the first couple of days after this physiologic inflammatory event (**Fig. 4**). Identification of onset of diestrus can be used to retrospectively define ovulation day. Whelping date can be projected as 56 to 58 days from diestrus onset or from 62 to 64 days from ovulation.

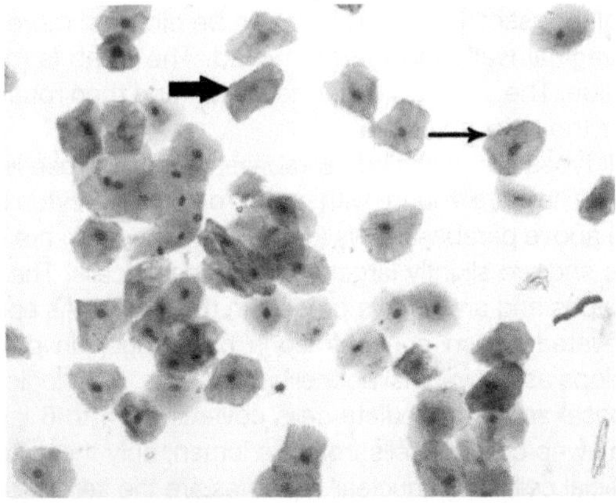

Fig. 2. Late proestrus vaginal cytology from a bitch. Note superficial epithelial cell (*small arrow*) and anuclear squamous epithelial cell (*large arrow*).

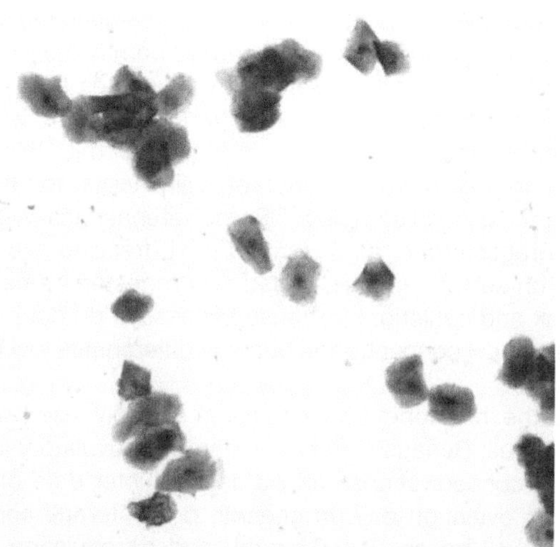

Fig. 3. Estrus vaginal cytology from a bitch. Note predominance of cells with no visible nucleus (anuclear squame cells).

Ultrasound of the Ovaries

Follicles can be seen on transabdominal ultrasound in bitches by experienced operators with good equipment, especially with serial evaluations of a given bitch. Ovulation is not readily defined by changes in sonographic appearance as follicles do not collapse at the time of ovulation and the CLs often have a cystic center.[15] This technique is not commonly used in clinical practice for determining stage of cycle in the bitch.

Hormone Assays

LH is the stimulus for ovulation in bitches. It is secreted pulsatilely, with a large, single peak associated with decline in serum estrogen concentrations in late proestrus or

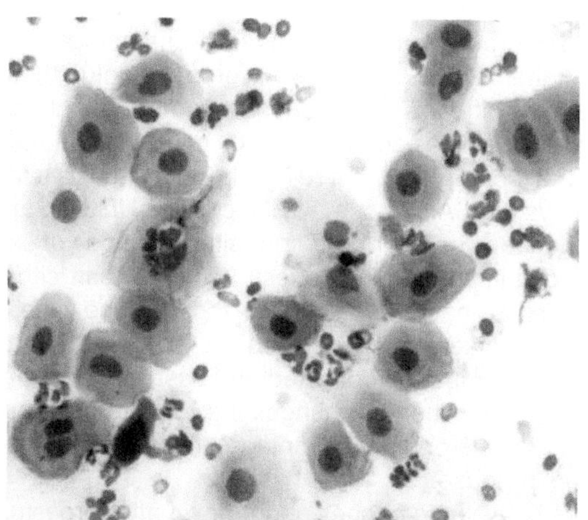

Fig. 4. Early diestrus vaginal cytology from a bitch. Note noncornified epithelial cells and presence of PMNs.

estrus. Ovulation occurs 36 to 50 hours later.[1] Direct measurement of LH is the most definitive diagnostic test available. Unfortunately, commercial LH assays are not readily available for the bitch and turn-around time makes their use impractical for clinical cases. In-house LH assays are intermittently available. Because duration of the LH peak is relatively short, daily testing is recommended; this is problematic for some owners due to logistics and cost of daily visits to the veterinarian for venipuncture and processing of samples.[15] Some veterinarians will circumvent this by drawing blood for progesterone, as described next, freezing extra serum, and then running LH assays on select samples, based on progesterone-based predictions of days of the LH peak and ovulation. In-house LH assays do not provide quantitative measurement of serum LH concentration but only differentiate low from high ($<$ or $>$1 ng/mL [3.1 nmol/L]).

Progesterone is the hormone assay most commonly used for assessment of ovulation date in bitches. Because bitches undergo preovulatory luteinization, rise in serum progesterone concentrations can be used to infer date of the LH peak and prospectively predict ovulation day. In general, progesterone concentration on the day of the LH peak will be about 2.0 ng/mL and on ovulation day from 4 to 10 ng/mL.[17] Some veterinarians prefer not to look at individual values but instead watch for a sudden increase in progesterone concentration by 3 ng/mL or more from one day to the next, denoting that as ovulation day. Some denote the first day progesterone concentration is 5 ng/mL or greater as ovulation day.[3] Finally, some veterinarians will look for an absolute value of progesterone at the time of breeding, with anecdotal reports of breeding optimized when progesterone is greater than 10 ng/mL or when progesterone is 15 ng/mL. The author is unaware of scientific studies documenting clinical significance of the latter method and prefers to use values to identify LH surge and ovulation day and to base timing of breeding on those values. It is generally accepted that one should not base all of one's decisions on a single blood sample as there is great variability between bitches. Collection of multiple blood samples over proestrus and estrus are required if any accuracy is expected in determining ovulation day using progesterone assay.

Progesterone can be measured using in-house assays or commercial assays. Commercial laboratories usually use either radioimmunoassay (RIA) or chemiluminescence assay (CA). These assays are quantitative. One study comparing RIA to CA demonstrated good correlation between the two when used to assay aliquots from the same sample. Progesterone concentrations in those samples assayed using CA were consistently higher by 0.69 ng/mL on average, a value those authors did not consider biologically significant.[18] It is valuable to note this difference in values by assay used, especially if samples are being run by more than one laboratory as a bitch is moved across the country for breeding. In-house assays are enzyme-linked immunosorbent assays (ELISAs); those available in the United States are semiquantitative, with various shades of color corresponding to ranges of serum progesterone concentration. Semiquantitative ELISA is less accurate than either RIA or CA. It is reported that ELISAs are inaccurate 85% to 89% of the time, with errors most commonly due to low values being misread as high.[19,20] Because the ELISA is semiquantitative, samples must be collected and assayed more frequently than with RIA or CA to ensure identification of changes in progesterone concentration significant for breeding timing. The primary advantage of ELISA assay is quick turn-around time as it can be run in-house.

The author prefers to evaluate bitches about day 4 after proestrus onset. If vaginal cytology is at least 60% cornified, blood is drawn for progesterone assay by RIA or CA. Samples are drawn every 3 to 5 days until values are suggestive of ovulation

(4–10 ng/mL). Sampling may continue past this time to ensure continuing increase in progesterone; one should never manage breeding based on only one progesterone value.[21] For natural service and artificial insemination (AI) with fresh semen or chilled semen, optimal breeding day is 2 days postovulation. Ideally, the bitch is bred at least twice, 2 and 4 days after ovulation. For frozen/thawed semen, which has decreased viability and so must be introduced when all ova are mature, insemination should take place 4 to 5 days after ovulation. Insemination too late after ovulation with any kind of semen is associated with decreased conception rate and increased embryo resorption, perhaps due to aging of DNA in the ova and subsequent errors in transcription or to asynchrony between embryologic development and the intrauterine environment.[22]

Miscellaneous Diagnostic Tests

Vaginoscopy can be used to gauge changes in the vaginal mucosa related to elevated circulating concentrations of estrogen. During anestrus, the vaginal epithelium is thin and the vasculature more readily visible, such that the mucosa is translucent red to pink and smooth. During proestrus, as estrogen stimulates vaginal edema and cornification, the mucosa will change from pink and billowy to white and sharp-edged. The sharp-edged, or crenated appearance, with subsequent loss of edema and wrinkling of vaginal folds, occurs approximately 2 days before ovulation.[15] This technique cannot be used alone to prospectively define day of ovulation.

Other measures that have been investigated include changes in electrical resistance across the vaginal mucosa, changes in glucose concentrations in vaginal fluid, change in progesterone concentrations in saliva, and ferning, or crystallization of vaginal fluid or saliva across glass slides (M.V. Root Kustritz and R. Davies, unpublished observations, 2003).[15,23] Although some correlations have been noted between these changes and physiologic events, none of the latter three techniques are sufficient to prospectively determine ovulation day.

ESTRUS INDUCTION

Because bitches cycle so infrequently compared to other species, there is great interest in inducing heat in this species. Induction of estrus may be used to treat pathologic anestrus, to make the bitch available for a given stud dog, to manage birth of pups at an optimal time of year, to ensure continuity of litter production for a breeding colony, to create reproductively similar dogs for research, to synchronize recipients for embryo transfer, or to teach canine reproduction.[7] No drugs are approved for estrus induction in bitches in the United States.

Bitches are more likely to respond to any estrus induction protocol if they are nearer the time of spontaneous proestrus onset.[24] This most likely is due to necessary changes in endocrinology in anestrus and also may be due to need for endometrial repair after the previous cycle.[7] The common therapies used for estrus induction are listed in **Table 2**.

General Management

It has been well demonstrated that bitches housed together will cycle together. This is called the *dormitory effect* and most likely is pheromonally based.[25] Bitches to be induced into proestrus are housed in close proximity with cycling bitches. This is noninvasive and inexpensive but consistency of this technique has not been reported. Other factors to consider when inducing estrus, especially in those bitches with pathologic anestrus, are general health and activity level. Very active bitches, such as hunting or show bitches, may not cycle due to alterations in body fat and associated

Table 2
Estrus induction protocols in dogs

Drug Type	Regimen(s) Described	General Success	General Concerns
Estrogen	DES; 5 mg once daily per os for 6–9 d or until proestrus induced	Few studies but good success reported, anecdotal reports variable	Split heat, lack of documentation about possible toxicity with repeated use
GnRH agonist	1. Ovuplant; 2.1 mg implant SQ 2. BioRelease deslorelin; 1.5 mg SQ	1. Good 2. Variable	1. Premature luteal failure, project variably available 2. Variable response
Dopamine agonist	Cabergoline Dostinex; 5 μg once daily per os for 30–40 days or until proestrus induced	Good	Expensive, difficult to dose for small bitches

changes in gonadotropin secretion. Bitches with systemic disease, such as hyperadrenocorticism, also may fail to cycle. Finally, some suggest that bitches with hypothyroidism may cycle less frequently. For this reason, it is valuable to perform a complete physical examination and routine blood work and to talk to the owner about management and activity level of the bitch before inducing estrus with any drug regimen.

Gonadotropins

The pituitary gonadotropins LH and FSH induce spontaneous proestrus, so one could hypothesize that treatment with these hormones could readily induce estrus. Unfortunately, protocols with these drugs have not been demonstrated to be successful. Treatment failure is associated with luteinization of follicles and ovulation failure, failure of implantation, and a shortened luteal phase.[3] Acute allergic response to LH was reported in 2 bitches.[7] A commercially available swine product (PG600; Intervet Schering-Plough, Summit, NJ, USA) contains 80 IU of equine chorionic gonadotropin (eCG) and 40 IU of human chorionic gonadotropin (hCG) per mL. Both eCG and hCG variably bind and activate LH and FSH receptors in bitches. In one study, injection of 5 mL of PG600 induced proestrus in 17 of 19 bitches and caused ovulation in 8 of 19; pregnancy rate was not reported.[7] Problems with use of PG600 for estrus induction in bitches include unpredictability of response, potential for allergic reactions to the large proteins contained in the product, and premature luteal failure.[7]

Estrogen

Estrogen priming occurs late in anestrus, making the ovary more responsive to pituitary gonadotropins. The goal of using estrogen for estrus induction is to increase responsiveness of the bitch to endogenous gonadotropins. Treatment with several different forms of estrogen has been described.[7] The most readily available regimen described is the use of diethylstilbestrol (DES; 5 mg per os once daily for 6–9 days or until onset of proestrus). Success rate in one study of 5 dogs was 100% for estrus induction, ovulation, and pregnancy in those bitches.[7] The author has had some bitches respond with a split heat, where they show signs of proestrus, go out of heat without ovulating, and then have a spontaneous heat within 4 to 6 weeks. Bitches have been successfully bred on that subsequent heat. There is nothing in the literature describing possible dangers of repeating treatment with DES to induce subsequent heat cycles; concerns about bone marrow suppression often are expressed anecdotally.

GnRH Agonists

GnRH agonists work by mimicking the normal increase in GnRH stimulation of gonadotropin secretion. GnRH is secreted pulsatilely and early work mimicked this pulsatile release by use of subcutaneous osmotic pumps. This technique, while successful, is not practical in clinics. Sustained administration of GnRH has been reported successful with some formulations. Concerns include failure to stimulate an adequate LH surge at the end of proestrus and premature luteal failure with prolonged administration.[7] Synthetic GnRH analogues vary in potency and efficacy.[7] Estrus induction is more successful in bitches with serum progesterone concentrations of <5 ng/mL.[26] GnRH agonists may be available either as subcutaneous implants or as depot injection preparations. The implant most commonly described for use in dogs is Ovuplant (Ayerst Laboratories, Guelph, Ontario, Canada), a product original designed for use in horses. A 2.1-mg implant is placed in the subcutaneous space, often in the vestibular mucosa just within the vulvar lips. Placement of the implant in an area from which it can be removed may be desirable.[27] Reported success rate for induction of proestrus within 2 to 9 days was 100%, with pregnancy rates varying from 40 to 67%.[7] This product is variably available in the United States. An injectable preparation is more readily available (BioRelease deslorelin; BET Pharmacy, Lexington, KY, USA). Subcutaneous injection of 1.5 mg one time was associated with variable success in induction of proestrus, with reported rates varying from 0 to 60%, and pregnancy rate also varying from 0 to 60%.[7]

Cabergoline

Cabergoline and bromocriptine are dopamine agonists that cause a decrease in serum prolactin concentrations and may be used to induce estrus in bitches. Bromocriptine is a human product and will not be described in detail. Cabergoline is a veterinary product (Dostinex; Pfizer, New York, NY, USA). The effect of cabergoline for estrus induction most likely is associated with its role as a dopamine agonist rather than in association with decline in prolactin.[7,14]

The standard dose regimen used for cabergoline is 5 μg/kg/day until proestrus is induced or for 30 to 40 days. A lower-dose regimen (0.6 μg/kg/day) was shown to be equally successful for estrus induction in one study.[28] The drug is available as a 0.5-mg tablet, which makes dosing difficult for small dogs. Dissolution in distilled water at room temperature to form a 10 μg/mL solution is described; this must be prepared daily and used within 15 minutes of preparation.[7] Compounding by dissolution into 1% acetic acid may create a more stable product.[29] Time until proestrus onset varies from 4 to 48 days.[28] Reported success rate for induction of proestrus is 80 to 100% and for pregnancy is 60% to 100%.[7] One reported side effect is change in coat color or texture.[7] This should be reversible as the hair follicles go through their normal cycle but will be of significant concern to owners of show bitches.

ESTRUS SUPPRESSION

Estrus suppression most commonly is effected in dogs in the United States by ovariohysterectomy. Gonadectomy is an effective and irreversible form of estrus control that may not be suitable in all situations and is associated with some detriments.[30] Similarly, immunologic means of contraception are being investigated for temporary or permanent estrus suppression in bitches.[31] This discussion will revolve around drug-based shorter-term estrus suppression in bitches.

Progestins

Progesterone-based products suppress estrus by negative feedback to the pituitary suppressing follicular development and subsequent secretion of estrogen, FSH, and LH.[32] Natural products exert significant progestogenic effects and are not commonly used. Synthetic forms of progesterone that have been used include megestrol acetate, medroxyprogesterone acetate, and proligestone. Megestrol acetate is administered at a low dose (0.55 mg/kg per os for 32 days) during anestrus or at a high dose (2.2 mg/kg per os for 8 days) during the first 3 days of proestrus. If used properly during anestrus, return to subsequent proestrus will be postponed for about 3 months. If used properly during proestrus, physical manifestations of proestrus and estrus, and breeding behavior will subside within days and the bitch will not ovulate on that cycle. Megestrol acetate was approved for use in bitches for estrus suppression but the commercial product is no longer available. Veterinarians can call prescriptions for megestrol acetate into human pharmacies. Medroxyprogesterone acetate is an injectable synthetic progestin. Severity of side effects and need for frequent readministration make this a less widely used drug. Proligestone is a synthetic progestin with few progestational properties, making it a more desirable injectable product. It is not available in the United States.

There are many reported side effects associated with use of progestins for estrus suppression in dogs. Synthetic products vary in their progestational properties.[32] It has been reported that if used as directed by the manufacturer, incidence of pyometra after treatment with megestrol acetate is about 0.8%.[31] Endometrial changes may be minimized by using drugs with less progestogenic activity and ensuring estrogen priming has not occurred.[32]

Progestins also may stimulate secretion of growth hormone with subsequent acromegaly, suppress the adrenal cortex, and suppress responsiveness to insulin, with subsequent diabetes mellitus.[32,33] Increased appetite and weight gain commonly are reported. Mammary stimulation with development of mammary nodules or neoplasia also has been reported.[3] Progestins may be teratogenic if administered to bitches early in pregnancy. Finally, localized reactions with hair loss and change in hair color have been reported in some bitches after use of injectable progestins.[32]

Androgens

Testosterone has never been approved for estrus suppression in bitches in the United States. Side effects include masculinization, clitoral hypertrophy, and aggression. Concerns have been expressed about long-term suppression of estrous activity in bitches treated with testosterone. Research results disagree as to whether treatment with testosterone interferes with subsequent ability to induce estrus in bitches.[34]

Mibolerone is a synthetic weak androgen that was approved for use in bitches for estrus suppression but is no longer available as a commercial product. The chemical may be available through compounding pharmacies. Therapy must be instituted at least 30 days before onset of the next proestrus. Dose varies with size of the dog, with dogs weighing less than 12 kg receiving 30 μg daily per os, those weighing 12 to 23 kg receiving 60 μg, those weighing 23 to 45 kg receiving μg mcg, and those weighing greater than 45 kg and all German shepherd dogs and their crosses receiving 180 μg daily. The drug is given continuously for up to 2 years and return to estrus after withdrawal of the drug averages about 70 days. Side effects include clitoral hypertrophy, exudation of creamy vulvar discharge, musky body odor and mounting behavior, and epiphora. This drug should not be used in Bedlington terriers.

GnRH Agonists and Antagonists

GnRH agonists suppress estrus by downregulation of hypothalamic and pituitary function. In postpubertal bitches with serum progesterone concentration less than 5 ng/mL, estrus may be induced first; this may be minimized by treating within 60 days of an ovulatory estrus, within 7 days of whelping, or following 7 days of progestogen therapy.[26,31] Treatment in prepubertal bitches is associated with prolonged estrus suppression.[26] Estrus suppression with subcutaneous implants containing either 4.7 or 9.4 mg of the GnRH agonist deslorelin suppressed estrus in 6 of 10 bitches in one study. Lower-dose implants must be replaced about every 4.5 months and higher dose implants more frequently than annually to be effective. No local side effects were noted.[35]

GnRH antagonists act by blocking effect of GnRH at the pituitary. Acyline is a drug that has been used to suppress estrus when implanted subcutaneously within the first 3 days of proestrus, with decrease in estrus signs within about 3 days and lack of ovulation on that cycle. Bitches returned to proestrus 20 to 25 days later.[36] Although this drug is not available in the United States, it would be most useful for bitches requiring very short-term suppression of estrus for travel or show purposes.

SUMMARY

Knowledge of the underlying endocrinology of the canine estrous cycle permits veterinarians to make the best possible recommendations to clients regarding management of their bitch's estrous cycle. Breeding management requires assay of progesterone to determine ovulation day. Estrus induction and suppression can be managed through drug or management schemes, with the client's understanding that no perfect protocols exist that would permit veterinarians to manipulate timing of estrus and ovulation with great accuracy.

REFERENCES

1. Concannon PW, McCann JP, Temple M. Biology and endocrinology of ovulation, pregnancy and parturition in the dog. J Reprod Fertil 1989;(Suppl 39):3–25.
2. Olson PN, Nett TM, Bowen RA, et al. Endocrine regulation of the corpus luteum of the bitch as a potential target for altering fertility. J Reprod Fertil 1989;(Suppl 39):27–40.
3. Concannon PW. Reproductive cycles of the domestic bitch. Anim Reprod Sci 2011;124:200–10.
4. Linde-Forsberg C, Wallen A. Effects of whelping and season of the year on the interestrous intervals in dogs. J Sm Anim Pract 1992;33:67–70.
5. Sokolowski JH, Stover DG, van Ravenswaay F. Seasonal incidence of estrus and interestrus interval for bitches of seven breeds. J Am Vet Med Assoc 1977;171:271–3.
6. Totton SC, Wanderler AI, Gartley CJ, et al. Assessing reproductive patterns and disorders in free-ranging dogs in Jodhpur, India to optimize a population control program. Theriogenology 2010;74:1115–20.

7. Kutzler MA. Estrus induction and synchronization in canids and felids. Theriogenology 2007;68:354–74.
8. Trigg TE, Doyle AG, Walsh JD, et al. A review of advantages of the use of the GnRH agonist deslorelin in control of reproduction. Theriogenology 2006;66:1507–12.
9. England GCW, Russo M, Freeman SL. Follicular dynamics, ovulation and conception rates in bitches. Reprod Dom Anim 2009;44(Suppl 2):53–8.
10. Concannon PW. Biology of gonadotrophin secretion in adult and prepubertal female dogs. J Reprod Fertil 1993;(Suppl 47):3–27.
11. Dore MAP. Structural aspects of luteal function and regression in the ovary of the domestic dog. J Reprod Fertil 1989;(Suppl 39):41–53.
12. Jeffcoate IA. Endocrinology of anoestrous bitches. J Reprod Fertil 1993;(Suppl 47):69–76.
13. McBride MW, Aughey E, O'Shaughnessy PJ, et al. Ovarian function and FSH receptor characteristics during canine anoestrus. J Reprod Fertil 2001;(Suppl 57):3–10.
14. Okkens AC, Kooistra HS. Anoestrus in the dog: a fascinating story. Reprod Dom Anim 2006;41:291–6.
15. England GCW, Russo M. Breeding management of the bitch. In: Bonagura JD, Twedt DC, editors. Current veterinary therapy XIV. Philadelphia: WB Saunders; 2008. p. 974–9.
16. Chandra SA, Adler RR. Frequency of different estrous stages in purpose-bred beagles: a retrospective study. Toxicol Pathol 2008;36:944–9.
17. Johnston SD, Root MV. Serum progesterone timing of ovulation in the bitch. In: Proceedings of Society for Theriogenology. San Antonio. Montgomery (AL): Society for Theriogenology; 1995. p. 195–203.
18. Chapwanya A, Clegg T, Stanley P, et al. Comparison of the Immulite and RIA assay methods for measuring peripheral blood progesterone levels in greyhound bitches. Theriogenology 2008;70:795–9.
19. Moxon R, Copley D, England GCW. Technical and financial evaluation of assays for progesterone in canine practice in the UK. Vet Rec 2010;167:528–31.
20. Manothaiudom K, Johnston SD, Hegstad RL, et al. Evaluation of the ICAGEN-Target canine ovulation timing diagnostic test in detecting canine plasma progesterone concentrations. J Am Anim Hosp Assoc 1995;31:57–64.
21. Seki M, Watanabe N, Ishii K, et al. Plasma progesterone profiles in beagle bitches with and without the whelping experience. Acta Vet Hung 2010;58:117–24.
22. Tsutsui T, Takahashi F, Hori T, et al. Prolonged duration of fertility of dog ova. Reprod Dom Anim 2009;44(Suppl 2):230–3.
23. Pardo-Carmona B, Moyano MR, Fernandez-Palacios R, et al. Saliva crystallisation as a means of determining optimal mating time in bitches. J Sm Anim Pract 2010;51: 437–42.
24. Verstegen JP, Onclin K, Silva LDM, et al. Effect of stage of anestrus on the induction of estrus by the dopamine agonist cabergoline in dogs. Theriogenology 1999;51:597–611.
25. Root Kustritz MV. Reproductive behavior of small animals. Theriogenology 2005; 64:734–46.
26. Trigg TE, Doyle AG, Walsh JD, et al. A review of advances of the use of the GnRH agonist deslorelin in control of reproduction. Theriogenology 2006;66:1507–12.
27. Kutzler M, Lamb SV, Volkmann D. Comparison between vestibular and subcutaneous insertion of deslorelin implants for oestrus induction in bitches. Reprod Dom Anim 2009;44(Suppl 2):83–6.
28. Cirit U, Bacinoglu S, Cangul IT, et al. The effects of a low dose of cabergoline on induction of estrus and pregnancy rates in anestrous bitches. Anim Reprod Sci 2007;101:134–44.

29. Wiebe VJ, Howard JP. Pharmacologic advances in canine and feline reproduction. Top Comp Anim Med 2009;24:71–99.
30. Root Kustritz MV. Determining the optimal age for gonadectomy of dogs and cats. J Am Vet Med Assoc 2007;231:1665–75.
31. Kutzler MA, Wood A. Non-surgical methods of contraception and sterilization. Theriogenology 2006;66:514–25.
32. Evans JM, Sutton DJ. The use of hormones, especially progestagens, to control oestrus in bitches. J Reprod Fertil 1989;(Suppl 39):163–73.
33. Kooistra HS, Okkens AC. Secretion of growth hormone and prolactin during progression of the luteal phase in healthy dogs: a review. Mol Cell Endocrinol 2002;197:167–72.
34. Phillips TC, Larsen RE, Hernandez J, et al. Selective control of the estrous cycle of the dog through suppression of estrus and reduction of the length of anestrus. Theriogenology 2003;59:1441–8.
35. Romagnoli S, Stelletta C, Milani C, et al. Clinical use of deslorelin for the control of reproduction in the bitch. Reprod Dom Anim 2009;44(Suppl 2):36–9.
36. Valiente C, Garcia Romero G, Corrada Y, et al. Interruption of the canine estrous cycle with a low and a high dose of the GnRH antagonist, acyline. Theriogenology 2009; 71:408–11.

Clinical Techniques of Artificial Insemination in Dogs

Chelsea L. Makloski, DVM, MS

KEYWORDS

- Artificial insemination • Transcervical insemination
- Transvaginal insemination • Canine • Dog
- Surgical insemination

Assisted reproductive techniques in the dog began in the 18th century when the first scientifically recorded artificial insemination was performed and produced 3 puppies.[1–3] Although this procedure had an early start, progress was slow to improve these methods. It was not until the mid-1900s that the first litter was produced using artificial insemination with frozen dog semen.[3] Since that time, the physiology and anatomy of the bitch have been studied extensively to develop techniques to determine ovulation timing, more successful transvaginal and transcervical insemination (TCI) methods, surgical procedures to deposit semen into the uterus and oviducts of the bitch, as well as other advanced techniques like embryo transfer and in vitro fertilization.

Reproduction in small animal veterinary medicine is rapidly expanding with a very high demand for the knowledge and skills necessary to produce litters, especially in the bitch. The following will aid clinicians in educating and assisting the backyard breeders as well as those more sophisticated breeders who may be having problems breeding the subfertile female or male.

OVULATION TIMING AND CYCLE MANAGEMENT

As clinicians, many of the "infertility issues" encountered in our patients, of any species, may stem from improper cycle management and ovulation timing. Before condemning a breeding female or male as an infertile animal, it is important to gather an accurate history of previous cycles, matings, illnesses, medications, and activities. This information will assist you in developing a plan for the next mating. Determining the type of breeding to be used—either natural mating, fresh semen, fresh chilled, or frozen semen—as well as the pregnancy rate of the male or semen to be used will also

The author has nothing to disclose.
JEH Equine Reproduction Specialists, 1030 Roland Road, PO Box 650, Whitesboro, TX 76273, USA
E-mail address: cmakloski.jehers@yahoo.com

Vet Clin Small Anim 42 (2012) 439–444
doi:10.1016/j.cvsm.2012.01.009 vetsmall.theclinics.com

assist in determining which insemination technique to use. Semen of lower quality or longevity will require more intensive tracking of the female's ovulation and possibly deposition of semen directly into the uterus or oviduct rather than the traditional vaginal deposition. Please refer to the article *"Managing the Reproductive Cycle in the Bitch"* by Root-Kustritz and colleagues in this edition for a more in-depth discussion of ovulation timing and breeding management.

BREEDING TECHNIQUES IN THE BITCH

Natural Mating

The goal of any breeding management program is to achieve the best conception rates and litter sizes as efficiently as possible. While this chapter is concentrating on artificial insemination, is would be remiss not to mention natural mating. This is generally the easiest and cheapest way to produce a pregnancy in most species, and in the bitch, there are 3 different strategies that may be applied.

The first strategy involves alternate-day breeding over the receptive period. Of the 3 strategies, this is the least expensive and involves the least amount of management. It works best if the male and female are owned by the same person or are housed on the same site and do not have a history of infertility. With this strategy, the male and female are generally housed separately and the female is brought to the male's domain once a day, both on leads, to observe for the presence of estrus behavior and mating if receptive.

The second strategy involves determining the approximate day of ovulation then breeding on days 4 and 6 or days 3 and 5 postovulation. The third strategy involves more intensive monitoring of ovulation and breeding. Conception rates in normal females bred once between 4 days before or 3 days after ovulation can be greater than 95%.[4] These strategies may be used if the male and female are not housed at the same location or male availability will only allow for 1 or 2 matings. These strategies can also be implemented with artificial insemination.[1]

It is important to bring the female to the male's territory to decrease some of the alpha female territorial behavior as this could impede the mating process. If the female exhibits estrus behavior but refuses mating or if the male is unable to mate a receptive female, then veterinary assistance should be sought with both patients examined for physical and physiologic abnormalities.

Transvaginal Insemination

Transvaginal insemination may be used when semen quality and bitch fertility are adequate, but natural mating cannot be accomplished due to either physical inability and behavioral problems. If transvaginal insemination is to be performed, it is necessary to have the appropriate equipment. Due to the varying breeds and sizes in the dog, it is important to select a sterile insemination catheter with adequate length to deposit the semen at the external os of the cervix. To do this, palpate the cervix in the caudal abdomen and estimate the distance to the vulva or estimate the distance from the costal arch of the rib cage to the vulva and divide the measurement by 2.[1] This distance will correlate with the length of the insemination pipette. In addition to the insemination catheter, a 6- or 12-mL air-tight syringe to deliver the semen, nonspermicidal lubrication, and exam gloves should also be used (**Fig. 1**).

To inseminate the bitch transvaginally, insert the pipette in the dorsal commissure of the vulva and direct it craniodorsally over the ischial arch. Next, direct it in a cranially. A gloved finger may be placed in the vulva to guide the passage of the pipette to the external os of the cervix. When proper placement of the pipette is

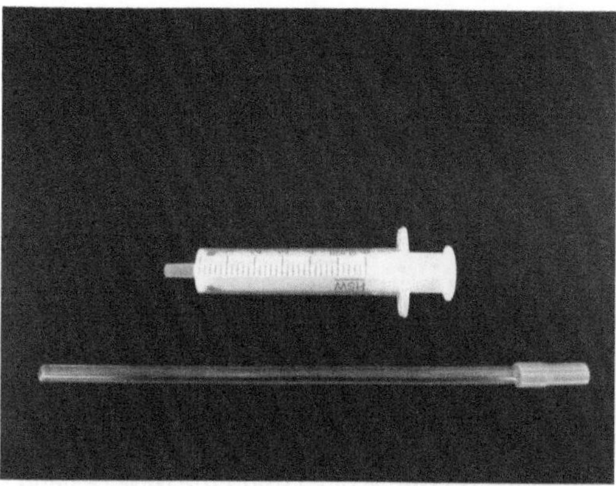

Fig. 1. Transvaginal insemination pipette and air-tight syringe used for insemination of the bitch.

achieved the semen is deposited into the vagina followed by 1 to 2 mL of air to flush the semen through.

The copulatory lock is bypassed during the insemination process and the hydrostatic pressure that it produces does not "push" the semen through the cervix. Due to this, it has long been recommended that the hindquarters of the bitch be elevated for 5 to 10 minutes after deposition of the semen to facilitate pooling of the semen at the external cervical os to increase pregnancy rates and litter sizes. In the past decade it has been shown that such a long duration may not be necessary as there was little effect in pregnancy rate and litter size by reducing hindquarter elevation time.[5]

Pregnancy rates with intravaginal insemination range between 60% and 95%. Such a large variation may be due to a number of reasons such as semen quality, the accuracy of ovulation timing, and the normality of the female reproductive tract. Litter sizes may vary as well for the same reasons.[5–8]

Transcervical Insemination

TCI has been recognized as a viable technique in canine reproduction. To perform this technique, there is a recognized "learning curve" and initial investments that can be discouraging. Despite this, TCI has become a popular and exceptional intrauterine insemination technique that removes the risks associated with anesthesia and surgery and can be used with fresh, chilled, and frozen semen.

There are 2 TCI techniques: the Norwegian method and the New Zealand endoscopic method. The least common technique, the Norwegian method, was first used for intrauterine insemination of foxes and was later adapted to the bitch. The equipment required for the Norwegian consists of a nylon sheath and metal catheter in 3 different sizes. This method requires skillful palpation and fixation of the cervix in the caudal abdomen. After achieving this, the metal catheter is manipulated through the cervix. Semen can then be deposited into the uterus.[9,10]

The second TCI technique (New Zealand endoscopic method) involves more specialized equipment but allows for visualization of the insemination process. With the use of a rigid endoscope and sheath (Storz Extended Length Cysto-urethroscope and sheath [KARL STORZ Veterinary Endoscopy America Inc, Goleta, CA, USA] or Minitube TCI Endoscope [Minitube of America, Inc., Verona, WI, USA]), light source, TCI catheter (Minitube TCI catheter), and optional camera and monitor (**Fig. 2**), TCI

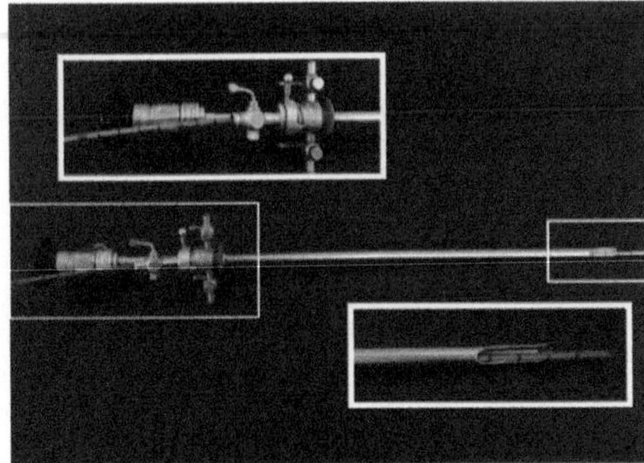

Fig. 2. Equipment required for TCI of the bitch using the New Zealand endoscopic method: Storz cysto-urethroscope, sheath, and TCI catheter.

can be achieved rapidly and with excellent results. The bitch is restrained in standing position. The endoscope is introduced and advanced through the vaginal folds. The dorsal median fold is the prominent landmark in the vagina and should be located and followed cranially. The external os of the cervix is in the center of a rosette of furrows on the dorsal aspect of the vagina. The catheter is advanced through the cervix with a twisting technique as far as it will go without force (approximately 2–3 cm).[11–13]

In addition to the learning process, TCI has other limitations that may be difficult to overcome such as the length of the vagina and the diameter of the paracervix, especially in small breed dogs. Visibility may be limited in some females with excess vaginal and uterine discharge. Identifying the cervical os may be difficult, as can cannulation of the cervix. Many of these obstacles can be overcome with patience and practice and can result in comparable pregnancy rates as seen in surgical insemination. Additionally multiple inseminations can be performed resulting in larger litter sizes.[7,8,14]

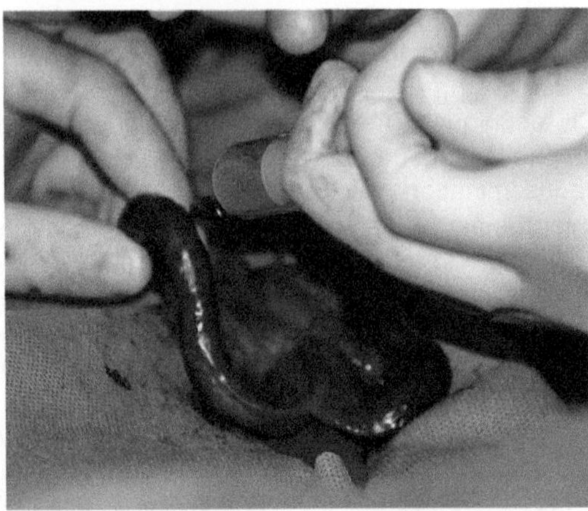

Fig. 3. Insemination of semen at the base of a uterine horn in a bitch via laparotomy.

Surgical Insemination

Surgical insemination is often useful in females as the surgeon can assess the uterus for pathology such as endometrial cysts, myometrial tone, and uterine wall thickness. Due to the unique physiology of the bitch, the endometrium is exposed to progesterone for extended periods of time, regardless of pregnancy status, and this accounts for progressive pathologic changes that result in cystic endometrial hyperplasia.[15–17] Changes in the endometrial lining can impact fertility in the bitch by diminishing the transport of semen to the oviducts, affecting conception, as well as interfering with placental attachment and embryologic and fetal health and growth.[17] The surgical approach for insemination should be considered in older females, subfertile females, females where uterine pathology is suspected, or females to be bred with a small or poor-quality dose of semen.

There are 2 types of surgical intrauterine techniques: the conventional and laparoscopic approaches. The conventional surgical insemination method is the most common technique used at this time as the incision is small, there is minimal manipulation, and many dogs return home within a few hours of surgery. For this method, the dog is anesthetized and placed in dorsal recumbency and a 2- to 3-cm incision is made through the skin and underlying linea alba. The uterine body and horns are isolated, and a sterile hypodermic catheter is introduced into the uterine lumen in the uterine body or base of either uterine horn (**Fig. 3**). The semen is then injected into the uterus. The surgeon can feel the uterus fill as the semen is inseminated. No incision is made into the uterus proper. The abdominal incision is then closed and the bitch is recovered from anesthesia.[18] This procedure has also been described in a lateral recumbency technique.

Laparoscopic intrauterine insemination has also been described with much success, but due to the additional costs for the equipment, additional training, increased setup time, and additional costs to the client, this technique has been slow to gain popularity. There does not appear to be a difference in pregnancy rates between surgical techniques with the rates nearing 100% when the female's reproductive cycle is properly managed, even in females with known fertility problems.[18,19]

One last surgical technique that has been described involves deposition of semen into the oviduct. This technique had been called intratubal insemination. This procedure is no more invasive than the laparotomy performed for surgical insemination and allows the clinician to inseminate lower numbers of sperm cells, but studies show a lower pregnancy rate than that encountered in intrauterine inseminations (surgical or TCI).[20]

SUMMARY

There are many instances where artificial insemination may be the best approach to achieve pregnancy in our canine patients, but it should never be substituted for poor management. It is important to consult with owners and thoroughly evaluate the bitch and stud dog and in the absence of the stud dog, the semen, to develop a breeding management plan. Knowledge and prior planning are the keys to success.

REFERENCES

1. Johnston SD, Root-Kustritz MV, Olson PNS, editors. Canine and feline theriogenology. Philadelphia: Saunders; 2001.
2. Dunlop RH, Williams DJ, editor. Veterinary medicine: an illustrated history. Philadelphia: Mosby; 1996.

3. Farstad W. Assisted reproductive technology in canid species. Theriogenology 2000; 53:175–86.
4. Holst PA, Phemister RD. Onset of diestrus in the Beagle bitch: definition and significance. Am J Vet Res 1974;35:401–6.
5. Pinto CR, Eilts BE, Paccamonti DL. The effect of reducing hindquarter elevation time after artificial insemination in bitches. Theriogenology 1998;50:301–5.
6. Pinto CR, Paccamonti DL, Eilts BE. Fertility in bitches artificially inseminated with extended, chilled semen. Theriogenology 1999;52:609–16.
7. Linde-Forsberg C, Forsberg M. Fertility in dogs in relation to semen quality and the time and site of insemination with fresh and frozen semen. J Reprod Fertil Suppl 1989;39:299–310.
8. Farstad W, Berg KA. Factors influencing the success rate of artificial insemination with frozen semen in the dog. J Reprod Fertil Suppl 1989;39:289–92.
9. Linde-Forsberg C. Achieving canine pregnancy by using frozen or chilled extended semen. Vet Clin North Am Small Anim Pract 1991;21:467–85.
10. Fougner JA, Aamdal J, Andersen K. Intrauterine insemination with frozen semen in the blue fox. Nordisk Veterinaermed 1973;25:144–9.
11. Wilson MS. Transcervical insemination techniques in the bitch. Vet Clin North Am Small Anim Pract 2001;31:291–304.
12. Wilson MS. Non-surgical intrauterine artificial insemination in bitches using frozen semen. J Reprod Fertil Suppl 1993;47:307–11.
13. Wilson M. Transcervical catheterisation techniques in the Bitch. Presented at: Society for Theriogenology. Baltimore (MD), December 4–6, 1998.
14. Linde-Forsberg C, Forsberg M. Results of 527 controlled artificial inseminations in dogs. J Reprod Fertil Suppl 1993;47:313–23.
15. Kim KS, Kim O. Cystic endometrial hyperplasia and endometritis in a dog following prolonged treatment of medroxyprogesterone acetate. J Vet Sci 2005;6:81–2.
16. De Bosschere H, Ducatelle R, Vermeirsch H, et al. Cystic endometrial hyperplasia-pyometra complex in the bitch: should the two entities be disconnected? Theriogenology 2001;55:1509–19.
17. Verstegen J, Dhaliwal G, Verstegen-Onclin K. Mucometra, cystic endometrial hyperplasia, and pyometra in the bitch: advances in treatment and assessment of future reproductive success. Theriogenology 2008;70:364–74.
18. Brittain D, Concannon PW, Flanders JA, et al. Use of surgical intrauterine insemination to manage infertility in a colony of research German shepherd dogs. Lab Anim Sci 1995;45:404–7.
19. Silva LD, Onclin K, Snaps F, et al. Laparoscopic intrauterine insemination in the bitch. Theriogenology 1995;43:615–23.
20. Tsutsui T, Hori T, Yamada A, et al. Intratubal insemination with fresh semen in dogs. J Vet Med Sci Jpn Soc Vet Sci 2003;65:659–61.

Current Advances in Gestation and Parturition in Cats and Dogs

Catherine G. Lamm, DVM, MRCVS[a,*], Chelsea L. Makloski, DVM, MS[b]

KEYWORDS

• Cat • Dog • Fetal monitoring • Gestation • Pregnancy

Normal gestation ranges from 57 to 72 days post breeding in the dog and 52 to 74 days post breeding in the cat, depending on the breed (cat and dog) and litter size (dog only).[1–5] The queen is an induced ovulator. The luteinizing hormone (LH) surge in cats occurs shortly after copulation with ovulation occurring approximately 24 to 40 hours later.[6–8] Unless copulation is directly observed, the exact time of ovulation in the queen is often difficult to determine. In the bitch, the variability of gestation length when calculated from the breeding date is due to the variable lengths of proestrus and estrus between individual animals. More accurate measurements of gestational length in the dog are based on the LH surge, with whelping occurring 64 to 66 days post LH surge.[9]

Approximately 5 days post breeding, the feline morulae enter into the uterus and the zona pelucida is shed 10 to 12 days post breeding.[1] Following transuterine migration, implantation occurs 12 to 13 days post breeding.[1] Heart beats are first detectable at days 16 to 25 post breeding.[1]

At 10 to 11 days following fertilization, the canine morulae replicates to form a 16-cell embryo.[10] From day 18 to 20, the blastocyst sheds the zona pellucida and the embryonic vesicle lengthens to 3 to 6 mm.[10] Transuterine migration throughout the uterine horns occurs during this period until implantation. Implantation of the canine embryo occurs at approximately 17 to 22 days post LH surge, and heartbeats are visible shortly after with ultrasound on days 23 to 25 post LH surge.[2,10–13] At roughly 4 weeks of gestation, reliable diagnostic tools become available to confirm pregnancy.[1,2]

The authors have nothing to disclose.

[a] School of Veterinary Medicine, University of Glasgow, Bearsden, Glasgow, G61 1QH, UK

[b] JEH Equine Reproduction Specialists, 1030 Roland Road, PO Box 650, Whitesboro, TX 76273, USA

* Corresponding author.

E-mail address: Catherine.Lamm@glasgow.ac.uk

Vet Clin Small Anim 42 (2012) 445–456

doi:10.1016/j.cvsm.2012.01.010 vetsmall.theclinics.com

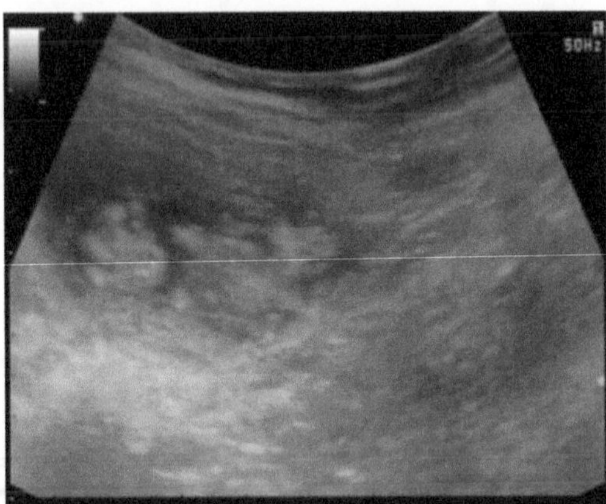

Fig. 1. Ultrasound image of a canine fetus approximately 38 days post LH surge.

PREGNANCY DIAGNOSIS

Ultrasound is one of the most sensitive and reliable forms of pregnancy detection in the bitch and the queen.[1] Pregnancy diagnosis should be attempted around 25 to 30 days post LH surge in the bitch.[2,12] The smallest fetal structures become apparent on ultrasound by skilled operators at 11 to 17 days post breeding in the queen and 17 to 20 days post LH surge in the bitch.[4,11,12,14] Pregnancy is more easily diagnosed by ultrasound 21 days following the LH surge in the bitch (**Figs. 1** and **2**).[2] Ultrasound is not always reliable in determining the number of fetuses present.[1,14]

Pregnancy diagnosis by transabdominal palpation is recommended at 22 to 30 days post LH surge in the bitch and at 21 to 25 days post breeding in the queen, when gestational sacs are palpable.[1,2,4,14] Occasionally, gestational sacs are palpable earlier but this is not as reliable. Between 30 and 45 days' gestation in the dog and at day 35 post breeding in the cat, the gestational sacs become flattened and until fetal

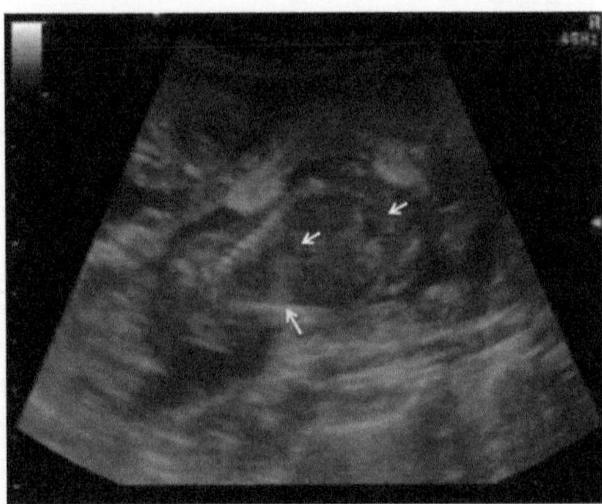

Fig. 2. Ultrasound image of a canine fetus approximately day 45 post LH surge. The urinary bladder and fetal stomach (*white arrows*) can be visualized and the fetal lungs (*yellow arrow*) are slightly more hyperechoic than the fetal liver.

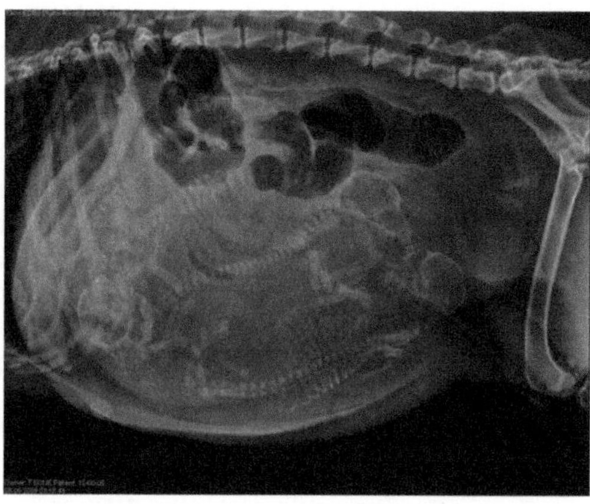

Fig. 3. Lateral radiograph in a dog with 5 term puppies. Distal extremities and teeth can be observed.

mineralization occurs, palpation may be difficult as the examiner must determine if uterine enlargement is due to pregnancy or uterine pathology.[1,4] Once fetal mineralization has occurred at days 42 to 45 in the dog and at days 38 to 40 in the cat, fetal skeletal structures are evident radiographically (**Fig. 3**).[1,2,4,12,14] Counting of fetal skulls on radiographs provides a relatively accurate estimation of fetal number.[4] Neither palpation nor radiographs can accurately assess fetal viability.

Serum progesterone concentrations are not reliable for diagnosis of pregnancy in either the bitch or the queen. This is due to prolonged luteal phases independent of pregnancy resulting in elevated concentrations of circulating progesterone.[2,4,15,16] In the queen, progesterone concentrations may become more reliable for pregnancy diagnosis at 20 to 30 days post breeding during which plasma concentrations peak at 15 to 30 ng/mL.[1,4,17] In the bitch, progesterone concentrations also increase with pregnancy but are rapidly metabolized by the placenta, resulting in similar circulating progesterone concentrations as nonpregnant bitches.[16] Progesterone metabolites can be measured in the feces of the bitch after day 25 and is diagnostic of pregnancy but is not routinely used.[16] After day 30, progesterone concentrations begin to decline.[1] Similarly, LH concentrations increase in both pregnant animals and nonpregnant animals in late diestrus.[2]

In contrast to progesterone, relaxin is specific to pregnancy in the bitch and queen.[4] As early as day 25, relaxin concentrations can be measured to diagnose pregnancy in the bitch with peaks as high as 4 to 5 ng/mL detectable at 40 to 50 days post LH surge.[2,4,10,11,15,16] An in-house relaxin assay is available (Witness Relaxin Test; Synbiotics, Kansas City, MO, USA) and allows for rapid results with serum or plasma. Similar to relaxin, prolactin can be used as an indicator of pregnancy as early as 35 days post LH surge in the bitch and 20 days post breeding in the queen.[11,15,17] Concentrations can be as high as 60 ng/mL in the bitch at the time of whelping.[4] However, serum prolactin concentrations are not as reliable as relaxin as they can be elevated in pseudopregnant animals. Elevated concentrations of follicle-stimulating hormone (FSH) can be seen as early as mid-pregnancy in the bitch.[18] This test is fairly expensive and is rarely used. Concentrations of 150 ng/mL or greater after 16 to 18 days post conception in the bitch are indicative of pregnancy. Nonpregnant females will have FSH levels less than 150 ng/mL.[2] These concentrations drop immediately following whelping.[18]

Increases in total estrogen concentrations can be detected in the urine of pregnant dogs 21 days post mating compared to nonpregnant dogs. It has been suggested that this assay could be made into a marketable in-house assay for veterinarians or owners, but to date this has not been developed.[11]

Some acute-phase proteins such as C-reactive protein and fibrinogen may be useful in diagnosing pregnancy in the bitch. Fibrinogen will increase at the time of implantation to approximately 280 mg/dL at 30 to 50 days' gestation, but unfortunately this protein is not specific to pregnancy as it may increase with other causes of inflammation.[2] C-reactive protein increases 20 to 25 days post ovulation in pregnant females but remains negligible in nonpregnant females. Levels will decrease rapidly if pregnancy is lost.[19] While measurement of C-reactive protein is a bit more reliable, it is not readily available in every laboratory.

Observation of behavioral changes is not an accurate way of diagnosing pregnancy in the bitch.[9]

MATERNAL CARE

Vaccination of the dam should occur prior to pregnancy and the administration of vaccines or other therapeutics should be limited during pregnancy.[2,4,12] Specific therapeutics are reported to have adverse affects in pregnant animals and are extensively listed in other locations so they will not be reviewed here.[2,4,12] Nutrition and exercise are critical during pregnancy.[4] Extra calories are not needed until the last 4 weeks of the pregnancy in the bitch and overfeeding is common.[2,4] A weight gain of 20% to 55% is considered normal and varies with breed.[4] In the bitch it is recommended that increases in bioavailable protein, fat, and trace nutrients be made in the later stages of gestation. Commercial puppy or growth diets containing 29% to 32% protein from an animal source, 18% fat, and 20% to 30% carbohydrates will generally meet the pregnant female's nutritional requirements.[20] While calcium requirements in the bitch are increasing during the last stage of pregnancy, it is important to avoid excessive calcium supplementation during this time as it has been determined this may predispose the bitch to eclampsia and dystocia. If calcium supplementation is necessary, this author prefers to start the female on oral calcium tablets after whelping. In contrast to the bitch, queens require a slow, steady increase in calorie intake from day 14 post breeding.[1,4,21]

PREGNANCY MONITORING

Monitoring of the dam can be used to follow any pregnancy but is specifically recommended in cases where owner and veterinary cooperation are necessary. This may occur in females where an elective cesarean section is desired. This may also include dams with a singleton pregnancy, giant breed animals with small litters, and dams with large litters and where there is concern of uterine fatigue or secondary uterine inertia or females with a history of dystocia. In addition to these, patients with high-risk pregnancies should be monitored closely. Patients with gestational diabetes mellitus, pregnancy toxemia, or those that have entered preterm labor that has been interrupted by tocolytic agents such as progesterone or terbutaline should have hormonal and ultrasonographic monitoring. The goal is to support the pregnancy to the earliest point when the neonates can survive an extrauterine environment without compromising the dam's health beyond recovery.

Physical Examination

Maternal heart rate increases with cardiac output and blood volume as pregnancy progresses.[2] As both dogs and cats are tetrapods ambulating on all 4 limbs, the gravid uterus distributes more weight throughout the abdomen, leading to slightly decreased gastrointestinal motility.[2] As pregnancy progresses, mammary gland development occurs, with onset of lactation beginning 2 weeks prior to or 7 days after parturition.[2]

Complete Blood Count and Serum Biochemistry Changes with Pregnancy

Pregnant bitches and queens may have a normocytic, normochromic anemia, with packed cell volumes dropping to 35% to 40% in bitches around 20 days post LH surge.[2,4,15] A mild neutrophilia can also be seen.[4] As mentioned, C-reactive protein and fibrinogen concentrations can be elevated but are not routinely tested.[4,10,22] Other serum biochemistry changes include decreased serum proteins, elevated lactate dehydrogenase, elevated cholesterol, and decreased blood urea nitrogen and creatinine.[2]

Ultrasound

Ultrasound is a safe and effective way to monitor fetal growth and viability. Fetal heart rate can be observed as early as 21 days[14] and becomes more reliable for diagnosis at 25 days post LH surge.[4] Fetal heart rates should be greater than 220 beats/min in the canine fetus and greater than 193 beats/min in the feline fetus.[1,23] Canine fetal hearts rates between 180 and 220 beats/min indicate moderate fetal distress and heart rates less than 180 beats/min indicate severe fetal distress.[23] Fetal bowel movements often accompany decreased heart rates in severe fetal distress.[23]

Fetal movement follows at approximately 31 days in the dog and 28 days in the cat.[1,14] Fetal age can be estimated based on the ultrasound measurements of the gestation sac, head, and body diameters as well as the crown–rump length. Fetal age in the bitch can also be determined by estimation of fetal maturation. The embryo proper can be visualized within the gestational sac by day 25 or 26 post LH surge and rests adjacent to the wall of the uterus. Fetal heartbeats may also be seen at this time. At days 27 to 28, the embryo moves away from the endometrial wall. The placenta appears zonary on ultrasound on days 29 to 31 with the edges curling inward on days 29 to 33. The fetal urinary bladder becomes evident between days 35 and 39, and the fetal stomach between days 36 and 39. The kidneys and eyes can be visualized on days 39 to 47, and the fetal intestines between days 57 and 63. The fetal lungs become more hyperechoic than the liver between days 38 and 42, and the liver becomes more hyperechoic than the other abdominal organs between days 39 and 47. Fetal intestinal peristalsis becomes evident between days 62 and 64. Fetal maturation along with fetal measurements can be used to obtain a more accurate estimation of fetal age. Calculations based on these measurements are outlined in **Table 1**. Ultrasound is an excellent tool in the diagnosis of fetal abnormalities. In dogs, intrauterine growth retardation is quantified by biparietal-to-abdominal diameter ratios of less than 2.[23]

Radiographs

Radiographs can also provide a rough estimate of gestational age but should not be the only tool used for determining readiness for birth. **Table 2** can be used to determine stage of pregnancy.[24] Abnormalities on radiographs, including gas pockets or disorganized fetal skeletons, may indicate fetal death with putrifaction or maceration, respectively.[4]

Table 1
Gestational age calculations based on ultrasonographic measurements in the dog and cat

Dog (±3 days)	
<40 days post LH surge[a]	Age = (6 × gestation sac diameter) + 20
	Age = (3 × crown–rump length + 27
>40 days post LH surge[a]	Age = (15 × head diameter) + 20
	Age = (7 × body diameter) + 29
	Age = (6 × head diameter) + (3 × body diameter) + 30
Cat (±2 days)	
>40 days post breeding[a]	Age = (25 × head diameter) + 3
	Age = (11 × body diameter) + 21

[a] Measurements are given in centimeters.

Data modified from Davidson AP, Baker TW. Reproductive ultrasound of the bitch and queen. Top Companion Anim Med 2009;24(2):55–63.

Progesterone Monitoring

For high-risk pregnant females, progesterone monitoring throughout pregnancy may be recommended. Progesterone is the hormone responsible for maintenance of pregnancy, and a decline in serum progesterone levels may indicate loss of corpra lutea possibly due to nutritional, environmental, traumatic, inflammatory, or idiopathic causes. In the face of decreased progesterone levels, females may enter preterm labor resulting in the loss of the litter. In some instances, preterm labor may be interrupted with tocolytic therapy such as exogenous progesterone supplementation or terbutaline.[25] Progesterone may also be used to determine onset of parturition in the bitch.[2]

Prepartum Rectal Temperatures

Prepartum rectal temperatures may be useful in predicting onset of whelping in the bitch. Progesterone, a thermogenic hormone, is responsible for the maintenance of

Table 2
Gestational age estimates based on visible radiographic structures

	Day of Detection After LH Surge	
Radiographic Structure	**Queen**	**Bitch**
Spherical uterine swellings	28–30	31–38
Ovoid uterine swellings	35	38–44
First evidence of mineralizations of the fetal skull	38–40	43–46
Scapula, humerus, and femur	38–40	46–51
Radius, ulna, and tibia	49	50–53
Pelvis and all ribs	43	53–59
Coccygeal vertebrae, fibula, calcaneus, and distal extremities	52–53	55–64
Teeth	56–63	58–63

Data modified from Lopate C. Estimation of gestational age and assessment of canine fetal maturation using radiology and ultrasonography: a review. Theriogenology 2008;70(3):397–402.

pregnancy in the bitch and it rapidly declines to less than 1 ng/mL 24 to 48 hours prior to parturition.[2] Decreases in the female's rectal temperature correlates with this decline in progesterone. Rectal temperatures in the bitch will abruptly decline at least 1 full degree 8 to 24 hours prior to parturition and are often less than 99°F. This "hypothermia" will persist for approximately 8 hours and then will increase back to euthermia at parturition.[26]

Tocodynometry

Tocodynometry involves the use of an external device that records uterine activity and fetal heart rates in pregnant bitches (WhelpWise; Veterinary Perinatal Specialties, Wheat Ridge, CO, USA). This service provides a rented uterine monitor and fetal heart rate Doppler and is generally started 3 to 5 days prior to due date unless otherwise recommended. The female wears the uterine monitor for 1-hour periods twice a day and the Doppler unit is used to monitor fetal heartbeats manually. The uterine monitor transmits data via a modem to a technician for interpretation of intrauterine pressures and fetal heart rates. This information can be shared with the attending veterinarian and can help diagnose fetal distress and differentiate eutocia from dystocia before clinically evident. Prompt intervention can decrease the incidence of fetal and maternal mortality.[27]

COMPLICATIONS DURING PREGNANCY

Maternal Factors

Innumerable maternal factors can contribute to pregnancy complications. Systemic disease and localized infection can play a role. Several diseases can develop during pregnancy as a consequence of the pregnancy itself and include pregnancy toxemia, diabetes mellitus, eclampsia, and hypertension.

Pregnancy toxemia is one of the most common complications of pregnancy in the bitch.[2] Bitches with inadequate carbohydrate intake, particularly those with large litters, have the potential to develop ketosis.[2] Clinical signs associated with pregnancy toxaemia are usually nonspecific. Ketonuria in the absence of a glucosuria is diagnostic. Diabetes mellitus is another complication of pregnancy and has similar, nonspecific clinical signs as pregnancy toxemia.[16] Diabetes can be differentiated from pregnancy toxemia by the presence of glucosuria with or without concurrent ketonuria.[2] Pregnancy toxemia and diabetes mellitus are both potentially life threatening to the dam and the offspring.

Eclampsia is caused by hypocalcemia and is more common in the dog than in the cat.[12] Hypocalcemia typically occurs post partum when the offspring begin to nurse and calcium demands are high; however, hypocalcemia can also occur during pregnancy. Clinical signs of eclampsia are nonspecific initially but may progress to muscle fasciculations or tremors, elevated rectal temperatures greater than 103.5°F, tetany, and, in severe cases, death. Calcium concentrations of less than 6.5 mg/dL in the dog and 6.0 mg/dL in the cat (ionized calcium $<$2.4 mg/dL in the dog) are diagnostic.[12] These values can vary depending on the laboratory and the reference values provided should be used to determine if the serum calcium concentrations are truly decreased.

Hypertension is a physiologic consequence of the cardiovascular alterations associated with pregnancy.[2] If complicated by preexisting cardiac disease, hypertension can affect the growth and survival of the offspring.[2]

Hypoluteoidism, or insufficient progesterone produced by the copora lutea, does not allow the bitch to maintain pregnancy. Luteal dysfunction may be primary (ovarian origin) or secondary (pituitary defect). This phenomenon has not been reported in the queen. Diagnosis requires documentation of low serum progesterone concentrations (<2 ng/mL) during diestrus. Blood samples should be monitored no less than once a week.[28–29] Caution must be used when making a diagnosis of hypoluteoidism as decreases in progesterone concentration is a normal physiologic response to fetal distress that may accompany premature labor or abortion from any cause.[2] Progesterone therapy including natural progesterone (4–6 mg/lb intramuscularly every 1–2 days) or progestational agents such as altrenogest (0.088 mg/kg/d per os) may be administered to maintain pregnancy. These therapies must be discontinued 1 week to 2 days before the anticipated whelping date to allow for normal parturition.[30] Owners should also be warned that progesterone therapy may cause masculinization of female pups if started prior to sexual differentiation is complete.[31] Decreased milk production has also been noted with this therapy, but this side effect is transient.[30]

Fetal Loss and Neonatal Death

Fetal death can occur in utero or during parturition. Delivery complications or periparturient infection can also lead to neonatal death.[2] Early embryonic death usually leads to fetal resorption and resumption of the estrus cycle, and pregnancy may not even be noted by the owner. Fetal death later in gestation results in expulsion of the fetus. Causes and diagnosis of fetal and neonatal death are discussed in an article in this issue by Lamm and colleagues.

NORMAL PARTURITION

Prior to the onset of parturition, the dam may exhibit altered activity levels, including nesting behaviors.[32] Parturition is divided into stages I to III. Stage I is characterized by synchronized uterine contractions, lasting about 6 to 12 hours. This results in dilation of the cervix. The dam may be restless, reclusive, anorexic, panting, or shivering. Vomiting may also occur. Stage II is characterized by complete cervical dilation and movement of the offspring into the birth canal. Stage III is when the fetal membranes pass. Stage II and III may overlap as some fetal membranes are passed with the individual offspring. Abnormalities in parturition can occur at any stage but most commonly occurring during stage II as a result of dystocia. Abnormalities in parturition and emergency interventions are covered in more detail in an article in this issue by Smith.

PREGNANCY TERMINATION

Pregnancy must be confirmed prior to attempts at termination. The safest and most effective way of termination pregnancy is ovariohysterectomy.[33] However, if the bitch or queen will be used for subsequent breeding, several therapeutics are available (though not all approved) for pregnancy termination in the United States. Therapeutics must be administered post ovulation and there is no single drug or drug combination that is 100% effective.[34] Some therapeutics are listed in **Table 3**. Therapeutics such as prostaglandins and prolactin inhibitors can be used in combination at slightly altered doses.[34] This allows for a synergistic effect resulting in higher efficacy with reduced side effects. If pregnancy termination occurs prior to day 40 in the bitch, fetal resorption is likely.[4] Serial ultrasound can be used to track resorption of fetuses less than 40 days of age.[14] Between days 41 and 65 post LH surge in the bitch, fetal expulsion is expected, and beyond days 50 to 55, the fetuses may be viable.[4] Hospitalization of the dam may be required following treatment in some cases to monitor for side effects and expulsion.[34]

Table 3
Therapeutics used for pregnancy termination in the bitch and queen

Estrogenic Compounds	Mechanism of Action		Side Effects	
	Inhibit embryo implantation		Cystic endometrial hyperplasia Pyometra Bone marrow aplasia Behavioral changes	
	Therapeutic	**Dose**	**Route**	**Comments**
	Estradiol cypionate	2–4.4 μg/kg (bitch), 0.125–0.25 mg/kg (queen)	IM	Given once, maximum dose is 1 mg
	Estradiol benzoate	2.5–5 μg/kg (bitch)	SQ	Given twice 2 days apart
	Tamoxifen	1.0 mg/kg (bitch)	Oral	Once daily for 10 days
Luteolytic Compounds	**Mechanism of Action**		**Side Effects**	
	Luteolysis		Prolonged treatment until progesterone concentrations drop below 2 ng/mL Reduction of intraestrus interval Tachypnea Hypersalivation Vomiting Diarrhea Ataxia Polyuria/polydypsia (dexametheasone)	
	Therapeutic	**Dose**	**Route**	**Comments**
	Dinoprost tromethamine ($PGF_{2\alpha}$)	50–250 μg/kg (bitch)[a]	SQ	Twice a day for 9 days
		500 μg/kg (queen, <30 dpb)[a]		2–3 times per day for 5 days
		500–1000 μg/kg (queen, >40 dpb)[a]		Once daily for 2 days
	Cloprostenol	1–2.5 μg/kg (bitch)	SQ	Once daily for 5 days
	Fenprostalene	20–50 μg/kg (bitch)	SQ	Once daily
	Dexamethasone	5 mg/kg (bitch)	IM	Twice daily for 5 days

(*continued on next page*)

Table 3
(continued)

Prolactin Inhibitors	Mechanism of Action		Side Effects	
	Luteolysis		Low efficacy in late pregnancy Similar to luteolytic compounds	
	Therapeutic	**Dose**	**Route**	**Comments**
	Bromocriptine	50–100 μg/kg (bitch)	SQ	Twice daily for 7 days
	Cabergoline	5 μg/kg (bitch)	Oral	Once daily for 7 days
	Metergoline	400–500 μg/kg (bitch)	Oral	Once daily for 5 days
Progesterone Inhibitors[b]	**Mechanism of Action**		**Side Effects**	
	Bind progesterone receptors or directly inhibit progesterone		Mammary gland development	
	Therapeutic	**Dose**	**Route**	**Comments**
	Mifepristone	2.5 mg/kg (bitch)	Oral	Twice a day for 4–5 days
		20–34 mg/kg (queen)	Oral	Single dose
	Aglepristone	10 mg/kg (bitch)	SQ	Once daily for 2 days
	Epostane	15–20 mg/kg	IM	Once

Abbreviations: dpb, days post breeding; IM, intramuscular; SC, subcutaneous.
[a] Lower doses can be used to reduce side effects.
[b] Currently not available in the United States.
Data from Root-Kustritz,[4] Wiebe and Howard,[12] Johnson and colleagues,[33] and Eilts.[34]

OVERT PSEUDOPREGNANCY (PSEUDOCYESIS OR PSEUDOGENETRA)

Each time a bitch enters estrus, she is designed to become pregnant. Many of the hormonal events that occur during pregnancy also occur during diestrus in the nonpregnant bitch. Prolactin is higher in bitches that have overt pseudopregnancies compared to other females that have covert pseudopregnancy. Signs of overt pseudopregnancy (pseudogenetra) include mammary development and lactation as well as behavioral changes such as nesting, mothering, and adopting inanimate objects.[35] Treatment is not generally recommended, but in severe cases bromocriptine (20 μg/kg once a day per os for 8–10 days) or cabergoline (5 μg/kg once a day per os for 5–10 days), both dopamine agonists, may be used.[36]

SUMMARY

Evaluation of the pregnant bitch or queen is best done approximately 4 weeks following the LH surge or post breeding, respectively. Diagnosis or pregnancy and fetal monitoring are best achieved through the use of ultrasound, although other methods are available. During this period, special attention should be made to the health of the dam, including appropriate nutrition and exercise. In cases of undesired pregnancy, termination can be achieved surgically or through the use of therapeutics.

REFERENCES

1. Johnston SD, Root Kustritz MV, Olson PN. Feline pregnancy. Canine and feline theriogenology. Philadelphia: Saunders; 2001. p. 421.
2. Johnston SD, Root Kustritz MV, Olson PN. Canine pregnancy. Canine and feline theriogenology. Philidelphia: WB Saunders; 2001. p. 66–104.
3. Okkens AC, Teunissen JM, Van Osch W, et al. Influence of litter size and breed on the duration of gestation in dogs. J Reprod Fertil Suppl 2001;57:193–7.
4. Root-Kustritz MV. Small animal theriogenology. St Louis (MO): Butterworth Heinemann; 2003.
5. Concannon P, Hodgson B, Lein D. Reflex lh release in estrous cats following single and multiple copulations. Biol Reprod 1980;23:111–7.
6. Shille VM, Munro C, Farmer SW, et al. Ovarian and endocrine responses in the cat after coitus. J Reprod Fertil 1983;69:29–39.
7. Sojka NJ, Jennings LL, Hamner CE. Artificial insemination in the cat (felis catus l.). Lab Anim Care 1970;20:198–204.
8. Tsutsui T, Stabenfeldt GH. Biology of ovarian cycles, pregnancy and pseudopregnancy in the domestic cat. J Reprod Fertil Suppl 1993;47:29–35.
9. Root Kustritz MV. Pregnancy diagnosis and abnormalities of pregnancy in the dog. Theriogenology 2005;64:755–65.
10. Concannon P, Tsutsui T, Shille V. Embryo development, hormonal requirements and maternal responses during canine pregnancy. J Reprod Fertil Suppl 2001;57: 169–79.
11. Concannon PW, McCann JP, Temple M. Biology and endocrinology of ovulation, pregnancy and parturition in the dog. J Reprod Fertil Suppl 1989;39:3–25.
12. Wiebe VJ, Howard JP. Pharmacologic advances in canine and feline reproduction. Top Companion Anim Med 2009;24(2):71–99.
13. Yeager AE, Mohammed HO, Meyers-Wallen V, et al. Ultrasonographic appearance of the uterus, placenta, fetus, and fetal membranes throughout accurately timed pregnancy in beagles. Am J Vet Res 1992;53:342–51.
14. Davidson AP, Baker TW. Reproductive ultrasound of the bitch and queen. Top Companion Anim Med 2009;24:55–63.

15. Concannon PW. Reproductive cycles of the domestic bitch. Anim Reprod Sci 2011;124:200–10.
16. Verstegen-Onclin K, Verstegen J. Endocrinology of pregnancy in the dog: a review. Theriogenology 2008;70:291–9.
17. Goodrowe KL, Howard JG, Schmidt PM, et al. Reproductive biology of the domestic cat with special reference to endocrinology, sperm function and in-vitro fertilization. J Reprod Fertil Suppl 1989;39:73–90.
18. Onclin K, Lauwers F, Verstegen JP. FSH secretion patterns during pregnant and nonpregnant luteal periods and 24 h secretion patterns in male and female dogs. J Reprod Fertil Suppl 2001;57:15–21.
19. Eckersall PD, Harvey MJ, Ferguson JM, et al. Acute phase proteins in canine pregnancy (canis familiaris). J Reprod Fertil Suppl 1993;47:159–64.
20. Moser E. Feeding to optimize canine reproductive efficiency. Probl Vet Med 1992;4: 545–50.
21. Wichert B, Schade L, Gebert S, et al. Energy and protein needs of cats for maintenance, gestation and lactation. J Feline Med Surg 2009;11:808–15.
22. Bunck CF, Mischke R, Gunzel-Apel AR. Investigation of the fibrinolytic system during nonpregnant and pregnant oestrous cycles of bitches. J Reprod Fertil Suppl 2001; 57:207–14.
23. Zone MA,Wanke MM. Diagnosis of canine fetal health by ultrasonography. J Reprod Fertil Suppl 2001;57:215–9.
24. Lopate C. Estimation of gestational age and assessment of canine fetal maturation using radiology and ultrasonography: a review. Theriogenology 2008;70:397–402.
25. Johnson CA. High-risk pregnancy and hypoluteoidism in the bitch. Theriogenology 2008;70:1424–30.
26. Concannon PW, Powers ME, Holder W, et al. Pregnancy and parturition in the bitch. Biol Reprod 1977;16:517–26.
27. Davidson A. Pariparturient problems in the bitch. Annual Meeting of the Socitey for Theriogenology. Montreal; 1997. p. 231–35.
28. Meyers-Wallen VN. Unusual and abnormal canine estrous cycles. Theriogenology 2007;68:1205–10.
29. Purswell BJ. Management of apparent luteal insufficiency in a bitch. J Am Vet Med Assoc 1991;199:902–3.
30. Eilts BE, Paccamonti DL, Hosgood G, et al. The use of ally-trenbolone as a progestational agent to maintain pregnancy in ovariectomized bitches. Theriogenology 1994;42:1237–45.
31. Mickelsen WD, Memon MA. Inherited and condenital disorders of the male and female reproductive systems. In: Ettinger SJ, Feldman EC, editors. Textbook of veterinary internal medicine. Philadelphia: WB Saunders; 1995. p. 1686–90.
32. Johnston SD, Root Kustritz MV, Olson PN. Canine parturition. Canine and feline theriogenology. Philidelphia: WB Saunders; 2001. p. 105-28.
33. Johnston SD, Root Kustritz MV, Olson PN. Prevention and termination of canine pregnancy. Canine and feline theriogenology. Philadelphia: WB Saunders; 2001. p. 168–92.
34. Eilts BE. Pregnancy termination in the bitch and queen. Clin Tech Small Anim Pract 2002;17:116–23.
35. Okkens AC, Dieleman SJ, Kooistra HS, et al. Plasma concentrations of prolactin in overtly pseudopregnant Afghan hounds and the effect of metergoline. J Reprod Fertil Suppl 1997;51:295–301.
36. Janssens LA. Treatment of pseudopregnancy with bromocriptin, an ergot alkaloid. Vet Rec 1986;119(8):172–4.

Clinical Approaches to Infertility in the Bitch

Robyn R. Wilborn, DVM, MS*, Herris S. Maxwell, DVM

KEYWORDS

• Infertility • Canine • Bitch • Estrus • Heat

Theriogenologists are often called on by clients and referring veterinarians to assist in evaluating fertility in bitches that have failed to produce a litter. The clinical approach to this dilemma in the canid is quite different than other species for several reasons. The inaccessibility of the female reproductive tract makes it quite challenging for the practitioner to gain useful diagnostic information. Palpation and ultrasonography are wonderful tools, but unless there is considerable pathology present or the examiner is quite experienced in scanning the female reproductive tract, the findings may be inconclusive. Samples for uterine cytology and biopsy can be obtained, but these procedures require a good deal of expertise and are much more invasive than in other species, sometimes necessitating general anesthesia and surgery. In addition to the inaccessibility of the female tract, the infrequency of the canine reproductive cycle makes it challenging to achieve a timely diagnosis. Owners and veterinarians are often frustrated with missed opportunities and the need to wait another 5 to 10 months to attempt another breeding.

Infertility is defined as the inability to conceive and produce viable offspring.[1] In litter-bearing species such as the bitch, subfertility may also be grouped with infertility to refer to instances in which litter sizes are smaller than expected. Although some of the causes discussed here can lead to pregnancy loss, this article will focus on the bitch that fails to conceive rather than reviewing causative agents for canine abortion. For more information on abortion in dogs, please see an article elsewhere in this issue.

When faced with a seemingly infertile bitch, it is necessary to spend a considerable amount of time taking a thorough history from the owner and handler. Each female has a unique set of circumstances and it is important to understand all aspects. Begin with the bitch's general medical history including previous illnesses, surgery, medications (particularly those used for estrus suppression), vaccination, and heartworm status. Once these data are collected, reproductive history should be addressed including dates of estrus and previous breeding attempts, method of insemination,

The authors have nothing to disclose.
Department of Clinical Sciences, College of Veterinary Medicine, JT Vaughan Teaching Hospital, Auburn University, 1500 Wire Road, Auburn, AL 36849-5522, USA
* Corresponding author.
E-mail address: wilborn@auburn.edu

Vet Clin Small Anim 42 (2012) 457–468
doi:10.1016/j.cvsm.2012.01.016 vetsmall.theclinics.com
0195-5616/12/$ – see front matter

pregnancy outcome including litter size, and whether ovulation timing was incorporated into the breeding management protocol. Finally, it is important to also obtain information about current environment, nutrition, housing, level of training, and breeding status of other dogs in the kennel.

Following the consultation with the owner and handler, a thorough physical examination should be performed. Examination of the external genitalia including digital examination of the vagina is indicated in appropriately sized bitches. Depending on the bitch's age and general health status, a minimum database may be warranted that includes a complete bold cell count, chemistry profile, and urinalysis. *Brucella canis* screening is recommend in all cases of canine breeding management, and particularly in cases of suspected infertility.[2–4] Further information on testing for *B canis* is covered in an article elsewhere in this issue.

Realizing that the reader's time is valuable, this article is divided into user-friendly headings to facilitate location of the section that best applies to your individual case. **Figs. 1** and **2** depict flow charts that are helpful in categorizing and managing suspected infertility cases. The reader is encouraged to review these algorithms prior to reading further to gain a broad understanding of some of the causes and contributing factors involved in the management of canine infertility.

Because reproductive histories often include vast amounts of information and circumstances, it is helpful to focus on simple questions that will serve to limit the list of differential diagnoses. For example, has the bitch been detected in estrus in the past 12 months? If so, then determine if the interestrus interval (IEI), or time from one estrus period to the next, is average (see **Fig. 1**). Normal IEI can be variable, but typically ranges from 5 to 8 months.[4] With this information, bitches can be further classified into one of the following categories.

IN ESTRUS WITHIN THE PAST 12 MONTHS; NORMAL INTERESTRUS INTERVAL

This category includes bitches having regular estrus periods at predictable intervals that have resulted in either no pregnancy or smaller than expected litter size. If the bitch has had predictable estrus periods with normal IEI, it is often helpful to focus on the most recent breeding attempts to determine why these efforts may have failed. It will be emphasized throughout that many cases of apparent infertility can be treated successfully with insemination of good quality semen at the proper time. Although this seems like a simple concept, appropriate breeding management is often overlooked as a mode of therapy for cases of suspected infertility.

Evaluation of Prior Breeding Management

The first aspect of breeding management to be considered, and the most common cause for suspected female infertility, is improper timing of insemination.[5–8] Many kennel managers routinely breed on days 10, 12, and 14 following the first sign of vulvar bleeding based on data indicating that these are fertile days for most bitches.[7,9,10] With proestrus lasting an average of 9 days, and estrus lasting an average of 9 days as well, this management protocol is often successful.[11] However, it should not be assumed that a bitch presented for infertility evaluation is average. In fact, it may be safer to assume that the bitch in question is NOT average. Many bitches that fail to produce a litter following a traditionally managed breeding (mated every other day on days 10–14) are NORMAL, but not AVERAGE. The reader is referred to an article elsewhere in this issue for a detailed review of the estrus cycle and ovulation timing, but it should be noted that some bitches linger in proestrus for up to 3 weeks or more before progressing into estrus.[12] Many of these bitches are reproductively normal but fall outside of the average range and may be perceived by

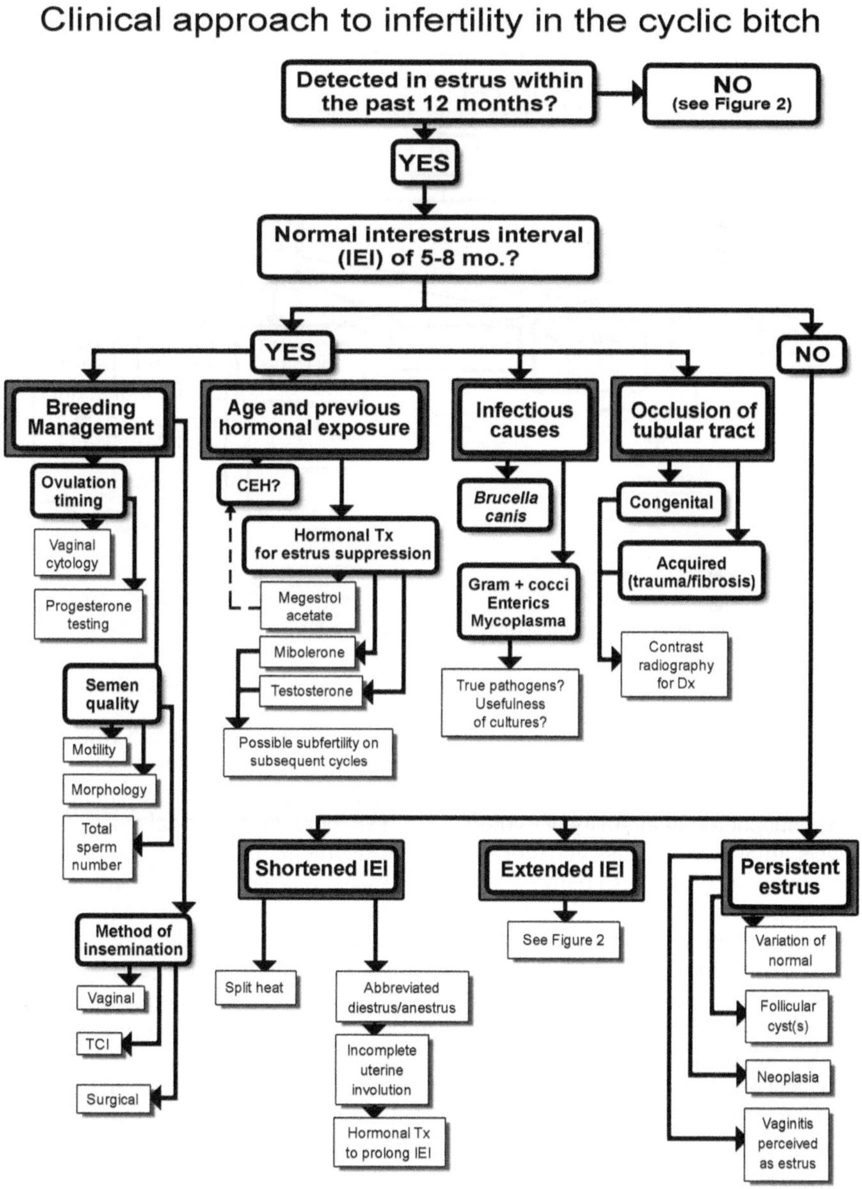

Clinical approach to infertility in the cyclic bitch

Detected in estrus within the past 12 months?
NO (see Figure 2)
YES
Normal interestrus interval (IEI) of 5-8 mo.?
YES
NO
Breeding Management
Ovulation timing
Vaginal cytology
Progesterone testing
Semen quality
Motility
Morphology
Total sperm number
Method of insemination
Vaginal
TCI
Surgical
Age and previous hormonal exposure
CEH?
Hormonal Tx for estrus suppression
Megestrol acetate
Mibolerone
Testosterone
Possible subfertility on subsequent cycles
Infectious causes
Brucella canis
Gram + cocci Enterics Mycoplasma
True pathogens? Usefulness of cultures?
Occlusion of tubular tract
Congenital
Acquired (trauma/fibrosis)
Contrast radiography for Dx
Shortened IEI
Split heat
Abbreviated diestrus/anestrus
Incomplete uterine involution
Hormonal Tx to prolong IEI
Extended IEI
See Figure 2
Persistent estrus
Variation of normal
Follicular cyst(s)
Neoplasia
Vaginitis perceived as estrus

Fig. 1. Algorithmic approach to infertility in the cyclic bitch.

the owners to be abnormal or infertile because they failed to conceive when mated on days 10 to 14. Errors in timing of insemination can easily be solved with ovulation timing. Running serial progesterone levels to determine a bitch's most fertile days often overcomes this common cause for apparent infertility and maximizes the chances for a successful breeding.

Semen quality and handling issues are a second area of breeding management that should be investigated when evaluating an apparently infertile bitch. This seems

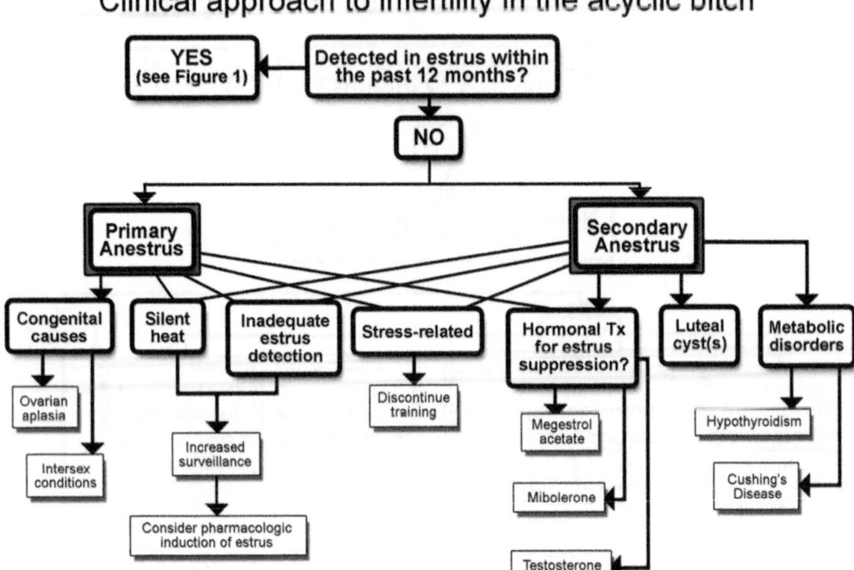

Fig. 2. Algorithmic approach to infertility in the acyclic bitch.

intuitive but is often overlooked. It is important to know if the male used was proven and if he has sired litters recently. A complete breeding soundness examination (BSE) is always desirable prior to breeding and is especially important when breeding bitches suspected of infertility or subfertility. A BSE includes a physical exam, motility analysis (total and progressive), morphologic assessment, and determination of total sperm number. All of these parameters can be measured easily with minimal training and equipment. Other ancillary testing may be indicated as well based on the individual patient. At the very least a simple subjective motility analysis, which takes only seconds and provides valuable information, should be performed and the results recorded at the time of insemination. This motility analysis is recommended with every assisted breeding including instances when cooled-shipped and frozen semen are used for breedings.

The final area of breeding management to be considered is the method of insemination. Vaginal inseminations are very commonly performed but achieve the best results with fresh semen of excellent quality. With fresh or cooled-shipped semen of marginal quality, and with all frozen semen breedings, an intrauterine insemination is recommended. This can be accomplished by catheterizing the cervix with the aid of vaginoscopy, a procedure commonly referred to as transcervical insemination. A second method that is commonly used for intrauterine deposition of semen is a surgical insemination. It is important to understand which insemination method was used during previous breeding attempts. For example, a vaginal insemination should not be used for frozen semen breedings as this yields reduced pregnancy rates.[13–15]

Influence of Age and Previous Hormonal Exposure

Once breeding management has been thoroughly reviewed, the practitioner should explore less common causes such as age and the potential influence of previous hormonal exposure (both endogenous and exogenous). Although cystic endometrial hyperplasia (CEH) will not be reviewed here in great detail, it should be mentioned as a contributing factor in infertility cases. Repeated exposure to estrogen followed by prolonged progesterone exposure during diestrus contributes to this disease process. This repeated hormonal exposure is coupled with the tendency of the diestrus canine uterus to respond to inflammation with cystic changes in the endometrial glands.[16–18] Bitches that are middle-aged to older often have some degree of CEH, and bitches that have never been pregnant are at increased risk.[19,20] This is often important in show or performance bitches that may not present for breeding until after their competitive career is complete and they are middle-aged. Diagnosis of CEH can be made via ultrasonography, direct palpation of the uterus during surgery, or uterine biopsy.[18,20,21] CEH should be suspected in any case when an older bitch fails to conceive following an appropriately managed breeding. Nulliparous bitches are at higher risk. In some instances, bitches with severe CEH may conceive but fail to produce a litter if the condition interferes with embryonic implantation.[8] Therapy options following diagnosis of CEH are limited. Several theriogenologists advocate the use of estrus suppression medications such as mibolerone in cases of CEH to prolong anestrus and allow the endometrium to regenerate.[19] However, mibolerone is not without its risks regarding future reproductive potential (see later). Anecdotal reports suggest that manual disruption of the cystic structures by "stripping" the uterine horns at the time of surgical insemination may be beneficial, but published reports and controlled studies are lacking.

Exposure to exogenous hormones may be a potential cause for infertility, particularly those commonly used for estrus suppression. Mibolerone, a synthetic androgen, is one of the most commonly utilized estrus suppression medications. This product was formerly marketed as Cheque drops (Upjohn, Kalamazoo, MI, USA) but is now available only from compounding pharmacies. Many bitches are placed on this drug while they are showing or competing and may remain on the drug for months to years. The label for the commercially available product indicated that the drug was for use in female dogs "not intended primarily for breeding purposes."[22] Studies by the manufacturer indicated interference with development of tertiary follicles and chronic exposure may induce endometrial atrophy. Fertility data on dogs that previously received mibolerone revealed a decreased conception rate on the first cycle after discontinuing the drug (76% vs 100% of controls).[22] For these reasons and due to anecdotal evidence, some theriogenologists advise against an expensive or invasive (ie, surgical) breeding on the first or even second cycle after discontinuing mibolerone (Society for Theriogenology Small Animal Listserv; November 2011).

Other hormonal therapies used for estrus suppression include testosterone (androgen) and megestrol acetate (synthetic progestin). Testosterone and other androgens likely have side effects similar to mibolerone, and progestins carry the added risk of induced uterine pathology including CEH. No drug therapy is without side effects, and owners should be cautioned that the fertility of estrus cycles following cessation of therapy may be suboptimal.

Infectious Causes of Infertility

Infectious agents may contribute to infertility in the cyclic bitch, and many owners of both bitches and stud dogs request vaginal cultures prior to breeding. Although vaginal cultures may be helpful in selected cases, interpretation of findings is difficult and the use of vaginal cultures as a diagnostic tool is reserved for situations where more common causes of infertility have been ruled out. Vaginal cultures should be obtained using a double-guarded sterile swab similar to those used in the mare.

Owners should be made aware that the canine vagina is not a sterile environment and that vaginal culture is expected to yield some growth.[23] Organisms commonly isolated from vaginal cultures of normal bitches include *Enterobacter* spp, gram-positive cocci, and Mycoplasma spp, among others.[20,24] Determining the pathogenicity of this bacterial growth can be challenging, however. In most cases when vaginal cultures are taken as a precaution or screening test in a seemingly healthy bitch, a light growth of mixed organisms is considered normal flora.[24] Heavy growth and pure culture of a single organism and repeated isolation of the same potential pathogen may implicate an infectious agent as a cause of infertility and warrant treatment. While the selection of antibiotic may be guided by culture results, timing and duration of therapy remain controversial. If vaginal cultures obtained from infertile bitches are accompanied by vaginal discharge, odor, or cytologic evidence of inflammation, then significant growth may truly indicate infection and treatment is warranted based on susceptibility. In any treatment protocol that is implemented near the time of insemination or during early gestation, teratogenic and embryotoxic effects should be considered. *B canis* is the only organism obtained from vaginal culture that is a definitive cause of infertility and is never considered normal flora.

Congenital or Acquired Occlusion of the Reproductive Tract

Although uncommon, occasionally the female tubular reproductive tract will lack patency due to congenital abnormalities or as a result of trauma or fibrosis. In either case, the bitch will usually continue to cycle normally but fail to conceive despite appropriate breeding management. These uncommon cases are best diagnosed via contrast radiography or exploratory surgery.

IN ESTRUS WITHIN THE PAST 12 MONTHS; ABNORMAL INTERESTRUS INTERVAL

Shortened Interestrus Interval

Bitches with a history of an abnormally short IEI generally fall into 2 groups: those having a split heat and those having an ovulatory estrus followed by an abbreviated diestrus/anestrus period. The more common of these 2 conditions is a split heat.

Split heats are often perceived by the owners to be 2 complete cycles that occur too close together (hence, a shortened IEI). However, a split heat occurs when the female shows signs of proestrus for several days but fails to progress to estrus and ovulation. The percentage of cornified cells seen on vaginal cytology will typically begin to decrease along with the signs of proestrus and progesterone concentrations never rise above 2.0 ng/mL. These bitches often have signs of proestrus again within 2 to 8 weeks and usually progress through a normal, fertile estrus at that time.[4,12,25]

Bitches with an abbreviated diestrus and/or anestrus period are those that return to heat less than 4 months following an estrus period with confirmed ovulation. An IEI of less than 4 months usually results in an infertile estrus due to incomplete uterine involution.[4] In order for the canine uterus to properly recover and involute following estrus, it must go through a diestrus period of progesterone influence for approximately 60 days before entering a state of anestrus. This obligatory anestrus period usually lasts around 90 days. Therefore, an IEI of 5 months or more is ideal for uterine involution and repair. Bitches with an abnormally short IEI can be treated with mibolerone (androgen) to keep them in a state of anestrus for a longer period of time, thereby allowing the uterus more time to undergo proper involution.[26]

Extended Interestrus Interval

Bitches that have had normal cycles previously but have experienced a prolonged period of time (>18 months) since their last heat are considered to be in a state of secondary anestrus.[27,28] Differential diagnoses for both primary and secondary anestrus are discussed in detail later in this article.

Persistent Estrus

Bitches that display signs of proestrus and estrus for longer than 30 days are considered by most owners to be abnormal. Before an infertility work-up is performed for this complaint, it should be emphasized that some normal bitches exhibit signs of proestrus for 28 days before progressing into estrus and a normal ovulation. As mentioned above in the section for *Breeding Management*, owners or managers may mistakenly breed several days ahead of ovulation in these bitches and inadvertently discontinue breeding prior to the fertile period. Vaginal cytology and progesterone testing should be performed in bitches suspected of experiencing a persistent estrus.[25] When normal bitches reach 90% to 100% cornification on vaginal cytology, progesterone should begin to rise within 7 to 10 days, signaling progression toward luteinizing hormone (LH) surge and ovulation and indicating a normal cycle.[12]

If cornification of vaginal cells persists for greater than 30 days with no corresponding rise in progesterone, ovarian pathology should be suspected. Cornification of vaginal epithelial cells confirms that the female is under the influence of estrogen, and failure to ovulate and progress to diestrus may be associated with estrogen-secreting follicular cysts or hormonally active neoplasia. Follicular cysts may be diagnosed via ultrasonography by an experienced operator, but serial observations may be required.[29–31] In cases of follicular cysts, medical therapy is aimed at inducing ovulation or luteinization using either gonadotropin releasing hormone (GnRH) or human chorionic gonadotropin (hCG).[32] Progesterone concentrations can be measured 7 to 14 days later to confirm ovulation or luteinization of persistent follicles or follicular cysts. Aspiration of follicular cysts via laparotomy has also been successful in at least one report.[33]

Cases of ovarian neoplasia may present as persistent estrus. In the case of ovarian neoplasia such as a granulosa cell tumor, signs of hyperestrogenism often persist manifested by an enlarged vulva, serosanguinous discharge, and the presence of cornified epithelial cells on vaginal cytology. If the hyperestrogenism continues for a prolonged period of time, endocrine alopecia and bone marrow suppression may also be seen.[32] If the hyperestrogenism is neoplastic in origin, attempts at inducing ovulation or luteinization using GnRH or hCG would be unsuccessful.[25] History and physical examination coupled with ultrasonography lead to many diagnoses, and it should be mentioned that spayed bitches with an ovarian remnant are also at risk. Hormonal testing may be necessary, and exploratory surgery is indicated in these cases to achieve both a diagnosis and cure.[34,35]

With a presenting complaint of persistent estrus, it should be noted that inexperienced owners can mistake signs of vaginitis for signs of estrus. It is not uncommon for male dogs to show interest in spayed or intact females when vaginitis is present. Although not well documented in the literature, this phenomenon occurs repeatedly per our conversations with referring veterinarians, and this interest from the male leads the owner to suspect that the female is in estrus. Serial vaginal cytology examinations are a quick and useful test to determine if the bitch is indeed under the influence of estrogen (evidenced by cornified epithelial cells) or has some degree of vaginitis (evidenced by neutrophils or other inflammatory cells).

NO ESTRUS DETECTED IN THE PAST 12 MONTHS

For bitches that have not been detected in estrus in the past 12 months, there are 2 major categories: primary anestrus and secondary anestrus. Primary anestrus is defined as having no detectable heat cycle by 24 months of age.[27] Secondary anestrus refers to bitches that have had previous estrus cycles but then cease cyclicity.[36]

Primary Anestrus

When presented with a female that has never been detected in estrus, one must determine whether this is truly a case of primary anestrus or whether the female has covert, or silent, heat cycles. **Failure to detect estrus is far more common than bitches that fail to display estrus signs.**

Silent heats/inadequate estrus detection

In some bitches, estrus may be difficult to discern (hence the term "silent heat"). Increased surveillance may be necessary to increase the chances of detecting the female in estrus, particularly if the bitch is housed in a kennel situation. A useful technique is to have the kennel manager blot the vulva twice weekly with a white paper towel to detect very subtle traces of serosanguinous discharge that may be present. This is especially useful in bitches that are very fastidious and those that are housed on raised grate-type kennel floors where small amounts of blood are not easily seen. The authors have seen this management technique become very effective in research colonies where raised floors and strict hygiene made estrus detection challenging.

Taking advantage of the "dormitory effect" may also improve the efficiency of estrus detection when bitches are group housed. Bitches housed together tend to come into estrus at the same time, and placing the seemingly anestrus bitch near other bitches with predictable estrus cycles can be a useful tool for improving estrus detection in females with silent heats.[4] When any females in the kennel are noticed to be in estrus, all females should be monitored very closely as many of them will follow suit.

Monthly progesterone (P4) testing can be done to determine if an unobserved estrus has occurred in a reportedly acyclic bitch. By testing P4 on a monthly basis, the practitioner can confirm ovulation by detecting a concentration of P4 that is typical of diestrus (15–90 ng/mL).[12] Elevated P4 in a bitch not observed in estrus indicates that estrus and ovulation occurred but that signs were not noticed. At that point, it can be expected that she would likely return to estrus in 4 to 6 months and should be monitored very closely around that time. This may be useful in convincing owners or kennel managers to invest more time in estrus detection for the cases of apparent anestrus. Increased surveillance from the owner or kennel manager often results in detection of the next estrus.

Owners often ask if pharmacologic agents can be used to induce a heat cycle, hoping for a "quick fix" to the problem based on their understanding of manipulation of the estrus cycle of horses and cattle. It is important that owners understand the differences in physiology between these species and the importance of the obligatory anestrus period in the canine, which allows the tubular reproductive tract to properly repair and prepare for a pregnancy. The authors strongly prefer the management practices mentioned above as a first step before resorting to pharmacologic induction of estrus. However, with owner consent and proper management by the practitioner, an estrus induction protocol can be a useful tool in confirming that the bitch is physiologically capable of completing an estrus cycle, indicating an intact hypothalamic-pituitary-gonadal (HPG) axis. Before initiating a pharmacologic approach, it is important to determine the current stage of the bitch's estrous cycle, to use the protocol as outlined, and to effectively communicate with the owner the pros and cons of using such agents to manipulate the cycle of the bitch.[37]

Stress-related anestrus

The lean body condition and elevated cortisol levels seen in some high-performing canine athletes can contribute to a breakdown of the HPG axis and an absence of cyclicity. Glucocorticoids suppress release of gonadotropins, particularly LH, which is required for ovulation.[38] Stress has long been suspected to play a role in bitches that experience ovulation failure during a seemingly normal estrus cycle, and for this reason it is often recommended to avoid shipping females until after a rise in progesterone has been documented indicating that the LH surge and ovulation have occurred.[11,39] Although not as well documented as in human medicine, the effects of stress on reproduction in the bitch are well grounded in empirical and anecdotal data. If this is suspected as a cause, the owner should be advised to take measures to reduce stress levels. For most bitches, this means ceasing training until an estrus cycle is detected. If this method results in a detectable estrus, the bitch should then not be allowed to resume training until after the puppies are weaned.

Hormonal therapy for estrus suppression

Medications used for estrus suppression were discussed previously in this article and will not be reviewed in detail here. However, it should be noted that these medications are commonly used in performance bitches and represent an important cause of anestrus. The owner should be questioned about the use of these and other common medications, such as glucocorticoids, that have been shown to have an effect on reproduction.[4]

Congenital causes

A less common but important group of conditions leading to primary anestrus are congenital abnormalities. Within this category are conditions such as ovarian aplasia and intersex conditions. In these types of congenital conditions, the animal is physiologically incapable of initiating and completing an estrous cycle. In most practical clinical situations, this is a diagnosis of exclusion once the methods mentioned above have failed to produce evidence of a normal cycle. Noninvasive diagnostics such as karyotyping can be performed if an intersex condition is suspected and the owner wishes to pursue testing for confirmation.

Secondary Anestrus

Cases in which bitches have previously had one or more normal estrus cycles and have not been detected in estrus for 10 to 18 months are referred to as secondary anestrus.[27,28] A history of normal estrus cycles rules out congenital causes in these cases. As mentioned earlier, failure to detect estrus is far more common than bitches that fail to display estrus signs, so inadequate estrus detection should be ruled out first in these cases. This is particularly important in a kennel situation and can often be remedied with the management practices detailed earlier. The next step should be to determine any management changes that have occurred in the household or kennel since the last time she was seen in heat. It is not uncommon for sporting and working dogs to cease cyclicity while in training due to stress, as discussed earlier.

Administration of medications, particularly those used for estrus suppression, can interfere with cyclicity. It is expected that most bitches will return to cyclicity anywhere from 2 weeks to 12 months of removing such therapy, so the owner should be advised to be patient.[4] It is best to allow the bitch to resume cyclicity on her own rather than attempting intervention with other hormonal therapies to induce estrus and hasten cyclicity.

Luteal cysts

Once the above causes have been ruled out, ovarian pathology should be considered, such as hormone-secreting ovarian cysts. Luteal cysts secrete progesterone and can cause the bitch to appear acyclic for several months. These can be seen ultrasonographically but are often difficult to distinguish from normal corpora lutea. Diagnosis of luteal cysts can be confirmed by documenting an elevation in progesterone of greater than 2.0 ng/mL for longer than the length of a normal diestrus (65 days).[9]

Metabolic disorders

Less commonly, metabolic conditions can lead to significant alterations in reproductive function and may be severe enough to lead to a state of secondary anestrus. Hypothyroidism may need to be addressed, particularly if indicated by clinical findings or requested by the owner. A complete thyroid panel is often recommended for any female with a history of infertility, particularly if she was previously considered reproductively normal and the owner now perceives that something has changed or a problem has developed over time. It remains unclear exactly what role hypothyroidism might play in secondary anestrus, and the degree to which it affects fertility.[40–43] Hyperadrenocorticism has also been shown to contribute to anestrus in the bitch, with over 75% of affected bitches in one study exhibiting a lack of cyclicity.[44] Both of these conditions are easily ruled out with diagnostic testing and most clients are willing to pay for quantitative data such as this to achieve a diagnosis.

REFERENCES

1. Blood DC, Studdert VP. Bailliere's comprehensive medical dictionary. Philadelphia: WB Saunders; 1998. p. 485.
2. Hollett RB. Canine brucellosis: outbreaks and compliance. Theriogenology 2006;66: 575–87.
3. Wanke MM. Canine brucellosis. Anim Reprod Sci 2004;82–83:195–207.
4. Johnston SD, Root-Kustritz MV, Olson PN. Clinical approach to infertility in the bitch. In: Kersey R, editor. Canine and feline theriogenology. Philadelphia: Saunders; 2001. p. 257–73.
5. Johnston SD, Olson PN, Root MV. Clinical approach to infertility in the bitch. Semin Vet Med Surg (Small Anim) 1994;9:2–6.
6. Zoldag L, Kecskemethy S, Nagy P. Heat progesterone profiles of bitches with ovulation failure. J Reprod Fertil Suppl 1993;47:561–2.
7. van Haaften B, Dieleman SJ, Okkens AC, et al. Timing the mating of dogs on the basis of blood progesterone concentration. Vet Rec 1989;125:524–6.
8. Freshman JL. Clinical approach to infertility in the cycling bitch. Vet Clin North Am Small Anim Pract 1991;21:427–35.
9. Davidson A. Current concepts on infertility in the bitch. Waltham Focus 2006;1321.
10. Fáy J, Mezö T, Solti L, et al. Comparison of different methods used for oestrus examination in the bitch. Acta Vet Hung 2003;51:385–94.
11. Johnston SD, Root-Kustritz MV, Olson PN. Breeding management and AI of the bitch. In: Kersey R, editor. Canine and feline theriogenology. Philadelphia: Saunders; 2001. p. 41–65.
12. Johnston SD, Root-Kustritz MV, Olson PN. The canine estrous cycle. In: Kersey R, editor. Canine and feline theriogenology. Philadelphia: Saunders; 2001. p. 16–31.
13. Nizanski W. Intravaginal insemination of bitches with fresh and frozen-thawed semen with addition of prostatic fluid: use of an infusion pipette and the Osiris catheter. Theriogenology 2006;66:470–83.

14. Thomassen R, Farstad W, Krogenaes A, et al. Artificial insemination with frozen semen in dogs: a retrospective study. J Reprod Fertil Suppl 2001;57:341–6.
15. Linde-Forsberg C, Strom Holst B, Govette G. Comparison of fertility data from vaginal vs intrauterine insemination of frozen-thawed dog semen: a retrospective study. Theriogenology 1999;52:11–23.
16. Chen YM, Lee CS, Wright PJ. The roles of progestagen and uterine irritant in the maintenance of cystic endometrial hyperplasia in the canine uterus. Theriogenology 2006;66:1537–44.
17. De Bosschere H, Ducatelle R, Vermeirsch H, et al. Cystic endometrial hyperplasia-pyometra complex in the bitch: should the two entities be disconnected? Theriogenology 2001;55:1509–19.
18. Cystic endometrial hyperplasia/pyometra complex. In: Feldman EC, Nelson RW, editors. Canine and feline endocrinology and reproduction. Philadelphia: Saunders; 1996. p. 605–18.
19. Verstegen J, Dhaliwal G, Verstegen-Onclin K. Mucometra, cystic endometrial hyperplasia, and pyometra in the bitch: advances in treatment and assessment of future reproductive success. Theriogenology 2008;70:364–74.
20. Johnston SD, Root Kustritz MV, Olson PN. Disorders of the canine uterus and uterine tubes. In: Kersey R, editor. Canine and feline theriogenology. Philadelphia: Saunders; 2001.
21. Bigliardi E, Parmigiani E, Cavirani S, et al. Ultrasonography and cystic hyperplasia-pyometra complex in the bitch. Reprod Domest Anim 2004;39:136–40.
22. Package insert for Cheque Drops (mibolerone). Kalamazoo (MI): The Upjohn Company; 1991.
23. Root Kustritz MV. Collection of tissue and culture samples from the canine reproductive tract. Theriogenology 2006;66:567–74.
24. van Duijkeren E. Significance of the vaginal bacterial flora in the bitch: a review. Vet Rec 1992;131:367–9.
25. Meyers-Wallen VN. Unusual and abnormal canine estrous cycles. Theriogenology 2007;68:1205–10.
26. Wanke MM, Loza ME, Rebuelto M. Progestin treatment for infertility in bitches with short interestrus interval. Theriogenology 2006;66:1579–82.
27. Johnston SD. Clinical approach to infertility in bitches with primary anestrus. Vet Clin North Am Small Anim Pract 1991;21:421–5.
28. Ovarian cycle and vaginal cytology. In: Feldman EC, Nelson RW, editors. Canine and feline endocrinology and reproduction. Philadelphia: WB Saunders; 1996. p. 526–46.
29. Hayer P, Günzel-Apel AR, Lüerssen D, et al. Ultrasonographic monitoring of follicular development, ovulation and the early luteal phase in the bitch. J Reprod Fertil Suppl 1993;47:93–100.
30. Poffenbarger EM, Feeney DA. Use of gray-scale ultrasonography in the diagnosis of reproductive disease in the bitch: 18 cases (1981-1984). J Am Vet Med Assoc 1986;189:90–5.
31. Wallace SS, Mahaffey MB, Miller DM, et al. Ultrasonographic appearance of the ovaries of dogs during the follicular and luteal phases of the estrous cycle. Am J Vet Res 1992;53:209–15.
32. Johnston SD, Root Kustritz MV, Olson PN. Disorders of the canine ovary. In: Kersey R, editor. Canine and feline theriogenology. Philadelphia: Saunders; 2001. p. 193–205.
33. Fayrer-Hosken RA, Durham DH, Allen S, et al. Follicular cystic ovaries and cystic endometrial hyperplasia in a bitch. J Am Vet Med Assoc 1992;201:107–8.
34. Sivacolundhu RK, O'Hara AJ, Read RA. Granulosa cell tumour in two speyed bitches. Aust Vet J 2001;79:173–6.

35. Pluhar GE, Memon MA, Wheaton LG. Granulosa cell tumor in an ovariohysterectomized dog. J Am Vet Med Assoc 1995;207:1063–5.
36. Infertility, breeding disorders, and disorders of sexual development. In: Feldman EC, Nelson RW, editors. Canine and feline endocrinology and reproduction. Philadelphia: WB Saunders; 1996. p. 619–48.
37. Verstegen JP, Onclin K, Silva LD, et al. Effect of stage of anestrus on the induction of estrus by the dopamine agonist cabergoline in dogs. Theriogenology 1999;51:597–611.
38. Kemppainen RJ, Thompson FN, Lorenz MD, et al. Effects of prednisone on thyroid and gonadal endocrine function in dogs. J Endocrinol 1983;96:293–302.
39. Goodman M. Demystifying ovulation timing. Clin Tech Small Anim Pract 2002;17:97–103.
40. Segalini V, Hericher T, Grellet A, et al. Thyroid function and infertility in the dog: a survey in five breeds. Reprod Domest Anim 2009;44(Suppl 2):211–3.
41. Panciera DL, Purswell BJ, Kolster KA. Effect of short-term hypothyroidism on reproduction in the bitch. Theriogenology 2007;68:316–21.
42. Johnson CA. Thyroid issues in reproduction. Clin Tech Small Anim Pract 2002;17:129–32.
43. Johnson CA. Reproductive manifestations of thyroid disease. Vet Clin North Am Small Anim Pract 1994;24:509–14.
44. Reimers TJ. Endocrine testing for infertility in the bitch. In: Kirk RW, editor. Current veterinary therapy VIII. Philadelphia: WB Saunders; 1983. p. 922–5.

The Problem Stud Dog

Cheryl Lopate, MS, DVM[a,b,*]

KEYWORDS

• Canine • Male infertility • Testicle • Spermatogenesis

Infertility may present as failure to produce pregnancy after mating, inability to mate or ejaculate, abnormalities of the spermiogram, clinical disease of the genitourinary tract, or physical defects in the reproductive tract. In some cases, infertility may progress slowly while in others onset of signs may be rapid. Male factor infertility is implicated in as many as 40% to 50% of cases of pregnancy failure.[1] Thorough history-taking, physical examination, semen collection, and evaluation, followed by appropriate diagnostics, will often yield a diagnosis. In some cases, treatment may be possible, but in many cases, no specific treatment is available, making careful and detailed breeding management of both the dog and bitch the mainstay of successful outcomes.

HISTORY

On presentation, a careful and thorough history is essential and should include general information, including age; kennel environment and living conditions including housing surface consistency (concrete, rocks, hardwood, etc); complete travel history; nutritional data including brand of dog food and any supplements administered; history of exposure to any person using topical steroid patches or creams; medications administered currently or previously; deworming history (dates and products used); prior health issues or concerns, including any immune mediated disorders; allergies; and genetic testing that has been completed along with the results of such testing.[2–5] Further detailed information about reproductive history should include: number of littermates (include number intact and if they have been used successfully for breeding); number of prior breedings; types of breedings performed; types of semen used either successfully or unsuccessfully; parity of bitches to which the dog was bred; age of bitches that were bred; if the bitches were confirmed pregnant and if so how; number of pups in each litter; chronologic history of semen evaluations and any history of hemospermia or pyospermia; prior diagnostics or treatments for infertility, including semen cultures; previous prostate exams (digital and ultrasonographic) and findings; history of urinary tract signs; history of

The author has nothing to disclose.

[a] Reproductive Revolutions, 18858 Case Road NE, Aurora, OR 97002, USA
[b] Wilsonville Veterinary Clinic, 9275 SW Barber Street, Wilsonville, OR 97070, USA
* Reproductive Revolutions, 18858 Case Road NE, Aurora, OR 97002.
E-mail address: lopatec1@gmail.com

Vet Clin Small Anim 42 (2012) 469–488
doi:10.1016/j.cvsm.2012.01.014 **vetsmall.theclinics.com**
0195-5616/12/$ – see front matter

constipation or ribbon-like stools; lameness problems, particularly hindlimb or back pain or injury; changes in scrotal size; any history of scrotal trauma or injury; and prior *Brucella canis* testing (type of test and dates performed).

PHYSICAL EXAMINATION

A complete and thorough physical examination should be performed.[2–5] This should start with general body systems paying careful attention to the nares and eyes for signs of abnormality in vision or olfaction; heart for arrhythmia or murmur; lungs; abdomen; pulse quality; peripheral lymph nodes; musculoskeletal system for signs of pain, swelling, lameness (paying careful attention to the lumbosacral spine and hind limbs); skin for signs of endocrine disease or atopy; and the neurologic system. A detailed examination of the reproductive tract should follow, including visual examination of the external prepuce and mucosal surface of the penis (both before and after erection) and a digital examination of the prostate for location (pelvic or abdominal), size, shape, symmetry, and pain. Examination of the scrotal contents includes examination of the scrotal skin for thickenings, alopecia, edema or masses; assessment of the vaginal cavity for fluid accumulation; palpation of the testicles for size, shape, tone, presence of masses or softening (focal or diffuse) and pain; and palpation of the epididymides and spermatic cords for enlargement, hypoplastic or aplastic regions, or pain. Measurement of total scrotal width can be performed with calipers or via ultrasonography.

SEMEN COLLECTION AND EVALUATION

Semen should be collected in the presence of an estrus teaser bitch whenever possible.[1,2,5,6] If a teaser is not available, the use of vaginal swabs from a bitch in heat, or estrus bitch urine may be applied to a non-cycling bitch. The dog's libido, ability to develop a normal erection, and mounting behavior, with character of pulsations and thrusting associated with ejaculation should be noted. The ease of which erection develops as well as the ability to develop and complete erection should be assessed. The prepuce should be cleaned prior to collection to remove any smegma present. The ejaculate should be fractionated if possible; but if not, then the approximate volume of each fraction should be noted. Fraction 1 is prostatic fluid, which clears the genitourinary tract of urine and debris prior to collection. As minimal an amount of fraction 1 as possible should be collected. The volume of fraction 1 is typically 1 to 4 mL. Fraction 2 is the sperm-rich fraction and may be 0.1 to 1.5 mL. Fraction 3 is prostatic fluid and may range in volume from 1 mL to 80+ mL. When prostatic disease is suspected, cytologic evaluation of a sediment of the third fraction will allow for characterization of this fluid.[3,7,8] Culture for aerobes, *Mycoplasma* spp and *Ureaplasma* spp may be performed if inflammation (acute or chronic) is suspected.

Semen evaluation should include volume, motility (total and progressive), velocity of forward progression, concentration/mL, total sperm/ejaculate, and morphology.[1,2,5,6] Sperm longevity can be evaluated every 24 hours after extending semen at a dilution of at least 3:1 in any of a variety of commercial extenders. Use of computer-assisted sperm assessment (CASA) for semen evaluation has been reported[1] and validated for canine sperm motility assessment while its use for evaluation of sperm morphology is still being investigated at this time.[9] Sperm concentration can also be determined with a hemacytometer or densimeter. Semen morphology is normally performed using stained slides (eosin-nigrosin, Wright-Giemsa) and oil immersion (×100) or with Formol-buffered saline or glutaraldehyde-fixed sperm and phase contrast or differential interference contrast microscopy. Morphologic abnormalities may be characterized as primary or secondary; compensable or noncompensable; and major or minor depending on the preference of the evaluator. Semen cytology can be performed with Wright-Giemsa stain if increased numbers of round cells are present in the ejaculate, in order to differentiate germ cells from white blood cells.[10] A normal spermiogram is expected to be greater than 70% progressively motile, with a velocity of greater than 4/5, having greater than 22 million spermatozoa per kilogram body weight in the total ejaculate, and greater than 70% morphologically normal.

ADVANCED SEMEN DIAGNOSTICS

When routine semen analysis fails to elucidate why a dog has infertility or subfertility, advanced diagnostics can be useful. Acrosome staining may indicate premature acrosome reaction or condensation of the acrosomal enzymes. The hypo-osmostic swelling test assesses the capability of the plasma membrane to transfer fluids across its surface normally.[1,11,12] Acrosome reaction testing and capacitation testing can be performed using fluorescent stains and exposure to calcium ionophore.[1,13,14] Electron microscopy may be used to detect ultrastructural abnormalities of the sperm head, acrosome, midpiece, or tail-piece.[1] Sperm chromatin structure assay evaluates DNA fragmentation and condensation.[1,15] Flow cytometry may also be used to detect sperm viability and abnormal cellular morphometry and DNA content when its use is combined with fluorescent staining.[1,13] Fluorescent microscopy can be used to assess DNA fragmentation and to identify specific chromosomal defects through the use of multiple assays.[1] Sperm penetration assays and hemi-zona assays evaluate the ability of the sperm to physically penetrate the zona pellucida and initiate interaction with the oocyte.[1] In vitro fertilization can be used to assess the ability of the sperm to not only penetrate the oocyte but also achieve fertilization.[1]

GENERAL ABNORMALITIES OF THE SPERMIOGRAM

Oligozoospermia is defined as an abnormally low number of spermatozoa in the ejaculate.[1–6] Less than 22 million sperm/kg body weight is considered abnormal. Asthenozoospermia is defined as a decreased number of progressively motile spermatozoa; having less than 30% to 50% progressively motile is considered abnormal.[1–6] Teratozoospermia is defined as an increased number of morphologically abnormal spermatozoa; having greater than 40% to 50% abnormal is considered abnormally high. Azoospermia is the absence of spermatozoa in the ejaculate.[1–6,16,17]

Dogs may present with a history of normal fertility followed by a decline in fertility, or they may have a consistent history of subfertility or infertility.[1–6,16–19] Subfertility or infertility may be defined as poor or low conception rates or small litter size despite good breeding management, decreased libido, or presence of the abnormalities of the spermiogram described earlier as found during breeding soundness examination. There may be a history of recent illness or fever in the last 2–3 months. There may be a history or suspicion of the potential use of anabolic steroids as a performance-enhancing drug or inadvertent exposure to exogenous steroid hormones via contact with estrogen or testosterone creams or patches used by owners, trainers, or handlers. There may be a history of bloody preputial drippings, hematuria, painful ejaculation, constipation or ribbon-like stools. In cases of asthenozoospermia, there may be a history of chronic or recurrent respiratory disease.[20–23]

Physical exam findings may include testes that are small, soft, firm, enlarged, or normal in size and consistency.[1–6,16–19] There may be enlargement or thickening of

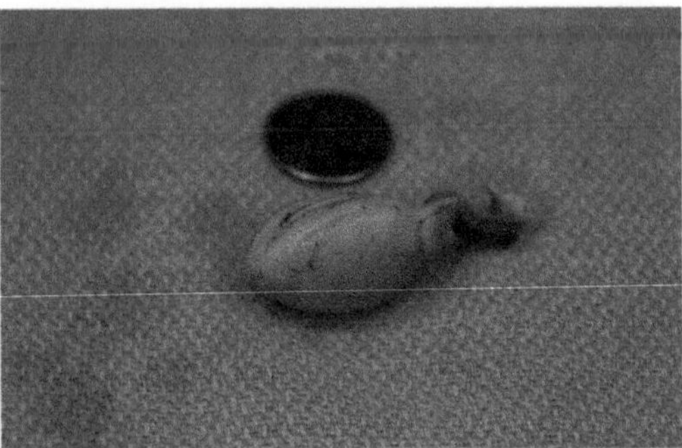

Fig. 1. Complete epididymal hypoplasia in a Boston terrier. The dorsal surface of the testicle (where the epididymis should be) is visualized here.

the epididymides or spermatic cords or obvious hypoplastic or aplastic regions (**Fig. 1**). There may be pain on palpation of the testes, epididymides, or cords. The scrotal skin may be thickened, lichenified, hyperpigmented, and/or alopecic. There may be palpable fluid within the vaginal cavity or the scrotum may be palpably edematous. The prostate may be enlarged, symmetrical or asymmetrical, painful or nonpainful. Dogs with primary ciliary dyskinesia may present with recurrent nasal discharge, cough, hydrocephalus, or situs inversus as well as asthenozoospermia.[20–23]

A list of differential diagnoses and possible diagnostic procedures for each of these spermiogram abnormalities are presented in **Table 1**. A list of possible treatment options for specific abnormalities of the spermiogram are presented in **Table 2**. A discussion of the specific conditions found in these tables follows.

SPECIFIC CONDITIONS CAUSING INFERTILITY

Prostatic Disease

Benign prostatic hyperplasia and hypertrophy (BPH)

BPH is the most common prostatic condition of the intact dog.[2–5,24,28,30] More than 50% of intact dogs with have signs of BPH by the age of 5 years and 80% will have signs by 6 years of age.[30] Hypertrophy and hyperplasia of the prostate occurs as a result of long-term exposure to the active metabolite of testosterone, dihydrotestosterone (DHT). BPH causes symmetric enlargement and increased vascularity, resulting in vascular leakage or hemorrhage into the gland. The blood is excreted through the prostatic portal system. Cellular swelling may result in formation of retention cysts, which may be single or multiple and of any size.

A history of sanguinous drippings from the penis is the most common presenting complaint.[2–5,24,28,30] This may occur only when exposed to bitches in heat, or it may occur intermittently or continuously. The blood may be fresh or digested (coffee-grounds appearance). Signs of urinary tract disease are uncommon. Constipation and production of a ribbon-like stool may occur once the prostate is markedly enlarged. Infertility may be another complaint. The prostate is typically uniformly enlarged, but smooth, symmetric, and nonpainful.[2–5,24,28,30] In some cases, enlargement may result in the gland being moved craniad into the abdominal cavity such that it cannot be reached by digital palpation. Complete blood count and serum chemistry are normal, unless acute infection accompanies the disorder. Radiography may reveal an enlarged soft tissue density in the caudal abdomen or cranial pelvic canal, just posterior to the bladder. In some cases, the bladder may be markedly enlarged due

Table 1
Differential diagnoses and diagnostic testing for abnormalities of the spermiogram

Spermiogram Abnormality	Differential Diagnoses	Diagnostic Testing
Oligozoospermia	• Scrotal overheating • Neoplasia • Prostatic disease • Infection of the reproductive tract • Testicular degeneration • Autoimmune orchitis or epididymitis • Pain, fear, or apprehension • Toxin or exogenous drug administration • Retrograde ejaculation[33,34] • Partial obstruction–sperm granuloma or spermatocele • Overuse • Collection of peripubertal dogs • Improper microscopic interpretation or operator error • Idiopathic	• History • Physical examination • Culture and cytology of third fraction or prostatic wash fluid and or sperm-rich fraction • Ultrasonography • Radiography (screening and contrast) • Serial semen evaluation in 60–90 days • Testicular aspirate or biopsy[36–39] • Testing for systemic illness as appropriate • Check urine for high sperm numbers • Baseline cortisol, ACTH stimulation, low-dose dexamethasone testing • Antisperm antibody testing • Drug testing (if known toxin) • Vitamin D concentration[25]
Azoospermia	All those for oligozoospermia plus: • Chromosome defects • Testicular hypoplasia • Sertoli cell only syndrome • Bilateral cryptorchidism • Hypopituitarism • Cushing or long-term steroid administration • Bilateral sperm granuloma • Following antineoplastic therapy, testicular sclerosing agents, or irradiation • Pain, fear, or apprehension (incomplete ejaculation) • Collection of prepubertal dogs	All those for oligozoospermia plus: • Karyotype • Seminal ALP >5000 U/L = ejaculation; <2000 anejaculation; 2000–5000 equivocal or partial ejaculation[40] • hCG stimulation testing • LH and FSH concentrations[41] • Testosterone, prolactin, and total estrogen concentrations
Teratozoospermia	• Testicular degeneration • Neoplasia • Scrotal overheating • Infection of the reproductive tract • Autoimmune orchitis or epididymitis[31,32] • Toxin or exogenous drug administration • Overuse • Abstinence fucosidosis[35] • Poor semen-handling techniques • Improper microscopic interpretation or operator error • Collection of peripubertal or geriatric dogs	• History • Physical examination • Ultrasonography (prostate and scrotal contents) • Testicular aspirate or biopsy • Culture of ejaculate and prostatic fluid • Testing for systemic illness as appropriate • Recheck semen evaluation in 60–90 days • Assay for alpha-L-fucosidase • Antisperm antibody testing • Drug testing (if known toxin) • Vitamin D concentration

(continued on next page)

Table 1 (continued)		
Spermiogram Abnormality	**Differential Diagnoses**	**Diagnostic Testing**
Asthenozoospermia	All those for teratozoospermia plus: • Collection using improperly washed or contaminated collection supplies • Excessive use of lubricants[30] • Prolonged exposure to latex, heat, or cold • Urine contamination • Abstinence • Immotile cilia syndrome–primary ciliary dyskinesia[20–24] • Reproductive tract infection	All those for teratozoospermia plus: • Evaluation of washing and drying protocols for reusable collection • Check all slide-warming equipment for defects • Electron microscopy of midpieces • Cultures of ejaculate and prostatic fluid

Data from Refs.[1–4,7,8,16,17,20–30]

to inadequate emptying. Retrograde cystourethrography may be necessary to illustrate prostatomegaly and to visualize the urethral architecture. There is often diffuse uptake of contrast from the urethra into the glandular tissue. The height of this uptake can be measured to assess severity of disease. Ultrasonography reveals a uniform hypoechoic to hyperechoic parenchyma with mild heterogenicity (**Fig. 2**). If there are intraprostatic cysts, symmetry between lobes may be distorted. The fluid within the cysts is typically anechoic.

Cytology of the prostatic secretions will have few white blood cells (WBCs) but may have many red blood cells (RBCs) or may be dark brown tinged due to lysed RBCs and digestion of the heme pigment.[7,8] If semen cannot be collected, prostatic massage or wash can be performed.[2–5,24,28,30] Prostatic fluid may be cultured (aerobic, *Mycoplasma* spp, *Ureaplasma* spp). If infection of the prostate occurs concurrently with BPH, cultures may be positive.[49] If prostatic fluid cannot be collected, culture and cytology can be obtained via ultrasound-guided aspiration cytology or biopsy.

Castration is the treatment of choice because it is curative.[2–5,24,28,30] Prostatic involution begins within days of castration and will be complete within 6 to 12 weeks. The size of the prostate at the time of castration dictates the length of time it will take to return to normal. Clinical signs may resolve well before involution is complete. In breeding dogs, treatment with finasteride at a dose of 0.1 to 1 mg/kg orally once a day is the treatment of choice. Finasteride is an 5α-reductase inhibitor and thus blocks conversion of testosterone to its active form, DHT, but only in the prostatic tissue.[50] It takes 2 to 3 months for the prostate to return to normal size with this medication. There is no effect on libido or semen parameters.[51,52] The amount of prostatic fluid may decrease significantly with long-term treatment, which will decrease the amount of fraction 3 produced, which may in turn affect natural breeding. For this reason, an alternate-day dosing schedule is usually administered once the prostate returns to its normal size.

Another treatment option is estrogen therapy.[2–5,24,28,30] Estrogens decrease gonadotropin secretion and thereby indirectly decrease testosterone production. Diethylstilbestrol (DES) at a dose of 0.2 to 1 mg/dog/day for 5 days is effective for up to 2 months. Estrogens may induce squamous metaplasia of the prostate so should not be used for long term treatment. Progestins may also be used but are not approved

Table 2
Treatment protocols described for abnormalities of the spermiogram in dogs

Medication	Dose Regimen	Condition Treated	Reported Response
Buserelin[42]	Once weekly × 3 doses 1 μg/kg SQ	Oligoasthenozoospermia	Increase in motility and total sperm numbers from wk 5–8 after first injection
hCG[43,44]	500 IU once weekly SQ × 9 wk; a single injection of 1000 IU IM	Oligospermia	Improvement in total sperm count starting 4 wk after onset of treatment and lasting 9 wk; total sperm numbers increased between 3 and 4 wk post treatment
GnRH agonist (Suprefact) ± hCG[45]	1 μg/kg SQ ± 500–1000 IU SQ once 4 wk after agonist treatment	Oligospermia	Improvement of total sperm numbers starting 4 wk after first treatment and lasting until 10 wk (improvement of morphology in 1 dog only); improvement of total sperm numbers at 2 wk after hCG and lasting 6 wk
Depot testosterone plus PMSG[46]	50 mg/dog testosterone + 250 IU PMSG IM q 2 wk × 3 doses	Oligospermia and asthenozoospermia	Increased sperm numbers and motility starting 1–5 wk after initiation of therapy and lasting 6–8 wk and slight improvement in tail defects from 2 to 6 wk after initiation
Fertirelin acetate (Conceral)[47]	400 μg IM	Asthenozoospermia Teratozoospermia	Motility increased between 2 and 8 wk after initiation of treatment; tail defects decreased from 3 to 7 wk after initiation of treatment
Aromatase inhibitor (AI), 4-androstene-4-ol-3,17-dione[48]	2 mg in cottonseed oil SQ	Azoospermia and increased estradiol-17β concentrations	Low sperm numbers present in 2 dogs with azoospermia

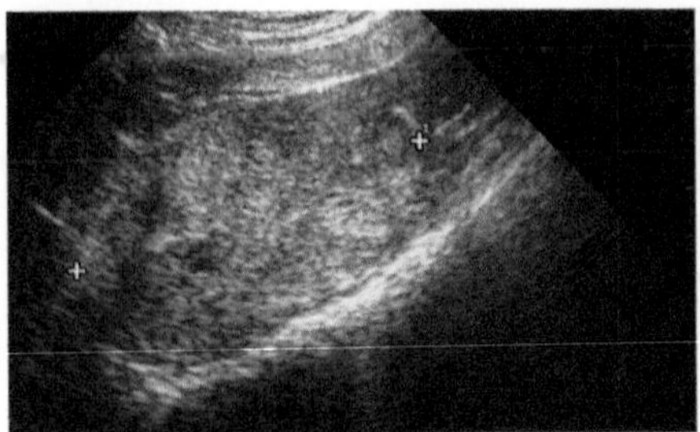

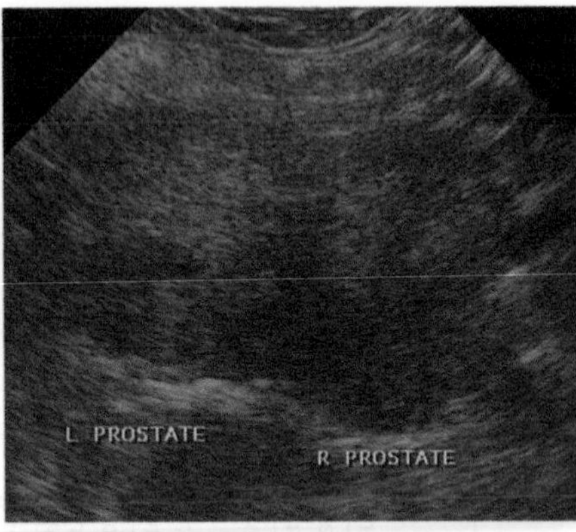

Fig. 2. Ultrasound image of a prostatic hyperplasia and prostatitis in a dog. This transverse image of the prostate demonstrates an asymmetric surface to the prostate gland with the right half being larger than the left. The echotexture is consistent with a mix of mild inflammation and hyperplasia.

for use in male dogs in the United States.[30] Megesterol acetate may be administered at a dose of 0.5 mg/kg daily for 4 to 8 weeks and results in reduction in prostate size within 1 to 2 months.[28] Alternatively, medroxyprogesterone acetate (MPA) can be administered subcutaneously at a dose of 3 to 4 mg/kg no more often than every 10 weeks.[28] Side effects include induction of diabetes mellitus or hypothyroidism and so these compounds are not recommended for treatment of BPH.

Delmadinone acetate (Tardak) is a progestagen with antiestrogenic and antiandrogenic characteristics.[53] It may be used at a dose of 1 to 2 mg/kg IM or SQ once and then repeated in 3 to 4 weeks if necessary. If inadequate response is seen in the first 8 days, a second dose can be administered at this time rather than waiting the standard 3- to 4-week waiting period. Side effects include decreased fertility and libido, lightening of hair color, hair loss, and exacerbation of diabetes. It is not currently available in the United States. Osaterone acetate (Ypozane) is another progestagen with antiandrogenic properties.[54] The typical dose is 0.25 to 0.5 mg/kg orally every day for 7 days. Side effects include a transient increase in sperm tail abnormalities (up to 6 weeks post treatment), exacerbation of hypoadrenocortism and diabetes mellitus, transient hepatic enzyme elevation (use caution in patients with hepatic disease), vomiting, diarrhea, polyuria/polydipsia (PU/PD), lethargy, and mammary gland hyperplasia.[54,55] Response is rapid with both these medications and effects last at least 4 to 6 months before signs will recur. Aromatase inhibitors have been described for use in treatment of BPH but have deleterious effects on semen quality and libido, so they should not be used in breeding animals.[56]

Prostatitis

Infection of the prostate is very common and is seen in all age groups from young dogs to older animals and is seen more commonly in intact dogs.[2–5,24,28,30] Presence of BPH, prostatic cysts, prostatic neoplasia, or squamous metaplasia may predispose to prostatic infection. Chronic prostatitis is more common than acute prostatitis and is more insidious in onset and clinical signs. Infection may occur from ascending infection from the urinary tract, preputial flora, epididymides or testes, hematogenously, or venereally (brucellosis).[57–59] The most common organism to infect the prostate is *Escherichia coli*,[49] but infection with a wide variety of aerobic and anaerobic bacteria and fungal organisms is possible.

In acute prostatitis, clinical signs may include swelling and edema of the prostate, fever (often >103°F), malaise, abdominal pain, vomiting, dysuria, stranguria, hematuria, tenesmus, constipation, obstipation, ribbon-like feces, and unwillingness to breed or pain on collection.[2–5,24,28,30] The prostate is typically painful but may be soft or firm and is usually swollen and asymmetric, particularly if abscessation occurs. The blood-prostate barrier is disrupted with acute prostatitis, which may lead to hematogenous spread of bacteria resulting in sepsis, disseminated intravascular coagulopathy, or multiorgan failure. Abscesses may rupture intra-abdominally resulting in peritonitis, sepsis, and rapid death. With chronic prostatitis, dogs are not typically systemically ill, but there may be signs of hematuria, tenesmus, constipation, obstipation, ribbon-like feces, and infertility and there may be a normal to enlarged, symmetric to asymmetric, nonpainful prostate, or there may be no signs at all.

With acute prostatitis, diagnostic testing may reveal pre- or post-renal azotemia, elevation in hepatic enzymes (particularly ALP), hypoproteinemia, electrolyte imbalance, leukocytosis with neutrophilia, often with a left shift, pyuria, and hematuria, while with chronic prostatitis blood work is typically normal.[2–5,24,28,30] Additional diagnostic testing may include abdominal radiography, retrograde cystourethrography, ultrasonography, and culture and cytology of prostatic wash or third fraction of the ejaculate.[2–5,7,8,24,28,30] Prostatic aspiration is cautioned when abscessation is suspected due to contamination of the needle tract with bacteria. Ultrasonography reveals a focal to diffuse heterogeneous echotexture with or without cavitating lesions filled with hyperechoic fluid. Infected areas tend to be hypoechoic to the normal parenchyma, although if mineralization is present, they may be hyperechoic.

Acute prostatitis requires aggressive therapy including intravenous fluids, nonsteroidal anti-inflammatory drugs (NSAIDs), and antibiotics.[2–5,24,28,30] Choice of antibiotics should be based on cytology and Gram stain until culture results are obtained. With acute prostatitis, the blood-prostate barrier is disrupted, allowing rapid penetration of most antibiotics into the gland regardless of prostatic fluid pH. With chronic prostatitis, choice of antibiotics is far more critical. Antibiotics with high lipid solubility, with high pK_a, and that are weakly alkaline will diffuse the most readily across the prostatic membrane. Good choices include trimethoprim-sulfa, clindamycin, chloramphenicol (high end of dose range required) and erythromycin. Alternatively, zwitterion antibiotics, like the fluoroquinolones enrofloxacin and ciprofloxacin, have multiple pK_a values, so they diffuse into the prostate regardless of the surrounding tissue and fluid pH.[60] Because enrofloxacin and ciprofloxacin are effective against most prostatic pathogens, they are frequently the first choice of antibiotics pending culture results for both acute and chronic prostatitis. With acute prostatitis, addition of amoxicillin, ampicillin, or amoxicillin plus clavulanate is often administered to ensure full gram-positive coverage. Fungal prostatitis may be treated with ketoconazole or itraconazole plus amphotericin B. Antibiotics should be continued a minimum of 4 weeks and while 8 to 12+ weeks is necessary for chronic cases or cases with abscessation.

Animals with concurrent BPH should be castrated or treated with finasteride.[2–5,24,28,30] Castration may help resolve prostatitis up to 4 to 5 weeks faster than antibiotic therapy alone. Prostatic abscesses may need to be surgically drained.

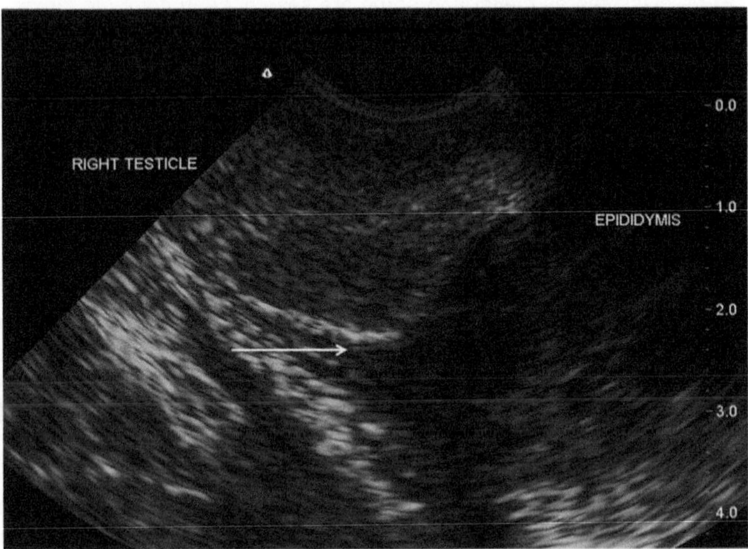

Fig. 3. Ultrasound image of a dog with epididymitis. Dilated tubular structures are located to the right of the testicle proper. The luminal diameter of the epididymis is at least 10 times its normal width. (*Courtesy of* Mary Stankovics.)

Infectious Orchitis and Epididymitis

Infectious orchitis/epididymitis is caused by bacterial, fungal, or viral infection that may ascend the urethra, descend from the prostate or bladder, arrive hematogeneously, or enter via puncture wounds.[2–5,16,17,24,26,39] It occurs more commonly in young dogs (average 4 years) and may be acute or chronic and are caused by a wide variety of bacteria, viral, and fungal organisms, such as *E coli, Klebsiella* spp, *Pseudomonas* spp, *Staphylococcus* spp, *Streptococcus* spp, *Brucella* spp, *Mycoplasma* spp, *Ureaplasma* spp, and *Blastomyces dermatitidis*.[8,49] Chronic infection results in atrophy and fibrosis.

Physical examination typically reveals enlargement, erythema, and pain in one or both epididymides, testes, or spermatic cords during the acute stage of infection.[2–5,16,17,24,26,39] If the disease is acute there may be fever, lethargy, hind-end lameness, scrotal pain, erythema and swelling, scrotal edema, and/or purulent preputial discharge. If the disease is chronic, there may be swelling or contraction of all or part of the scrotal contents, which is typically nonpainful and firm. Semen collection will often reveal pyospermia, but in acute cases, animals may be too painful to ejaculate. Sperm granuloma may be associated with this inflammation, either primarily or secondarily, as a result of fibrosis, local inflammation, and sperm agglutination.[61,62]

Diagnostics include culture and cytology of the ejaculate and ultrasonography.[2–5,16,17,24,26,39] Ultrasound typically reveals a heterogeneous architecture with inflamed areas being hypoechoic to the normal parenchyma. There may be areas of abscessation within the parenchyma or epididymides, which appear as anechoic or hyperechoic fluid-filled areas (**Fig. 3**). In more chronic cases, hyperechoic foci (with acoustic shadowing) may be apparent due to fibrosis or mineralization in the testicular interstitium (**Fig. 4**). Doppler ultrasound may reveal increased blood flow to the affected side during acute disease. Aspiration cytology or biopsy of these areas will reveal neutrophilic inflammation. Aspiration

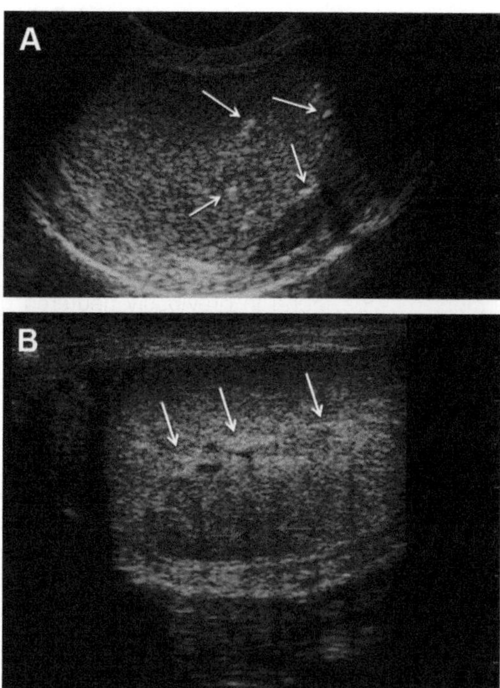

Fig. 4. Ultrasound image of testicular degeneration in the dog. (*A*) Mineralization is evident by the pinpoint hyperechoic foci (*white arrows*). (*B*) Fibrosis and mineralization is indicated by the wide hyperechoic bands (*white arrows*). Note the acoustic shadowing (*red arrows*).

of fluid pockets is possible and this fluid should be submitted for cytology and culture. Cytology ± Gram staining should be performed on any collected fluid or aspirates to help identify the initial choice of antibiotics. If no samples are available for cytology, either enrofloxacin or ciprofloxacin is a good first choice pending culture results, since they are both effective for a majority of reproductive pathogens. All dogs presenting with scrotal enlargement should be tested for brucellosis (see another article by Libby Graham elsewhere in this issue).[2-5,16,17,24,26,39,57–59]

If the process is unilateral, hemicastration is effective and may salvage the remaining testicle.[2–5,16,17,24,26,39] Removal of the affected side may prevent local extension of the infection and prevent ascension up the genitourinary tract. If the animal is bilaterally affected and future breeding is desired, then appropriate antibiotics should be administered long term (4–12+ weeks). If response to therapy is not immediate, castration should be considered. NSAIDs and cold packing of the scrotum are recommended to reduce inflammation and swelling, but should be used with caution long term, due to the potential deleterious effects on spermatogenesis.[63–66]

Sexual rest should be provided until resolution of clinical signs and return to spermatogenic function has occurred.[2–5,16,17,24,26,39] Return to normal semen quality can be expected in no less than 60 days and may take several months depending on the degree of injury to the remaining tissues. After unilateral castration, a compensatory hypertrophy of the remaining testicle may occur, bringing total sperm numbers up to two-thirds of the prior total. Prognosis for an affected testicle to return to normal is poor since spermatogenesis is often permanently affected. Relapse or ascension to the prostate or bladder is common.

Scrotal Overheating

Heat-related oligospermia and teratozoospermia may be present in tropical regions or during the hottest summer months in some countries due to the testes being maintained continuously at an elevated temperature.[2–5,16–18,24,26,27] The testes are meant to be maintained approximately 1.5°F lower than core body temperature (range 99°–101.5°F). Other causes of derangements in testicular temperature include excess scrotal insulation in obese dogs; hydrocele or hematocele; orchitis; epididymitis; scrotal edema from trauma, insect bite, and hypersensitivity reactions, chemical or contact irritants; testicular neoplasia; fever; varicocele; or ischemic insult. Treatment involves addressing the primary cause of the overheating insult. Return to normal spermatogenesis may take 60 to 180 days.

Autoimmune Orchitis and Epididymitis

Autoimmune orchitis/epididymitis occurs as a result of breakdown of the blood-testis barrier from trauma, infection, ischemia, or toxin exposure.[32,33] It has been linked in some cases to autoimmune thyroiditis and has been shown to be hereditary at least in some cases. Most cases present with a history of prior fertility followed by subinfertility or infertility. The progression may be slow to rapid and the condition eventually results in testicular degeneration or azoospermia. Diagnosis is based on history, semen evaluation with worsening oligo- or azoospermia and teratozoospermia, antisperm antibody testing, and testicular cytology or histology.[10,37–40] There is no treatment but the disease may be slowed or semen quality improved transiently with hormone therapy.[42–49,67]

Testicular Degeneration

Testicular degeneration may occur primarily from senescence or secondarily following trauma, inflammation, toxin exposure, autoimmune orchitis/epididymitis, overheating insult, neoplasia, infarct, obstruction, or endocrinopathy.[2–5,10,16,19,24,26,37–48,67,68] Clinical signs will vary depending on the primary cause of the degeneration. Diagnosis is based on physical examination, semen evaluation, ultrasonography, endocrinology (elevated follicle-stimulating hormone, prolactin or estradiol concentrations), cytology, and/or biopsy (see **Fig. 4**). Treatment of the primary disorder should be initiated as early in the disease process as possible. Remission in signs may be noted initially, but this is a chronic, progressive condition, so eventually sperm production will diminish and terminate. Hormone therapy may help slow the progression of signs.

VASCULAR INSULT OR INFARCT

This may occur as a result of a breakdown of the blood-testis barrier, trauma, inflammation or autoimmune disease and may occur unilaterally or bilaterally in dogs of any age.[3,10,16,24,26,37–40] Testicular degeneration is common sequelae to infarct and may occur in both testicles due to derangement of thermoregulation or may occur only in the affected testicle. Semen evaluation reveals teratozoospermia and/or oligozoospermia. Physical exam and diagnostics may lead to the diagnosis of other immune disease, with the testicular lesions being found incidentally. Diagnostics include ultrasonography, revealing a triangular hypoechoic lesion (**Fig. 5**), and testicular aspiration, revealing hypospermatogenesis to Sertoli cell only syndrome in

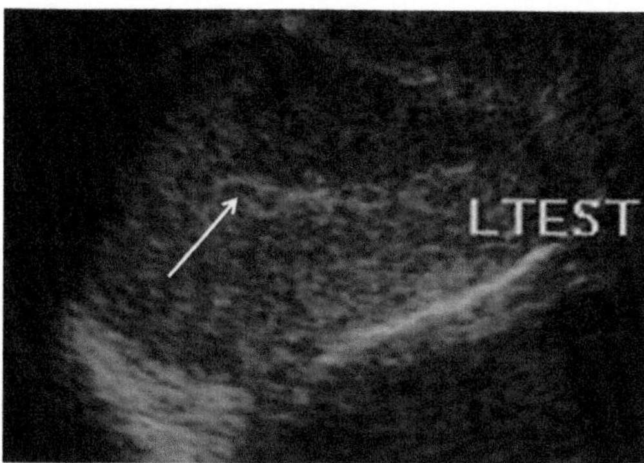

Fig. 5. Ultrasound image of a testicular infarct in a dog. Note the hypoechoic lesion at the dorsum of the testicle (*arrow*). It is triangular in shape, consistent with ischemic insult.

the affected area. Treatment is hemicastration, but the risk of a similar infarct occurring in the remaining testicle is high. Semen evaluation 60 to 90 days after surgery should show return some return of normal spermatogenesis if it is going to occur. Hormone therapy may encourage some improvements in spermatogenesis, albeit temporarily in many cases.[42–48,67]

Scrotal Trauma or Dermatitis

Trauma or dermatitis may result from physical injury, environmental trauma, chemical trauma, external parasites, allergic reactions, infectious agents, immune-mediated disorders, or sperm granuloma.[2,3,27,57–59] Scrotal trauma or dermatitis typically results in thickening of the scrotal skin, which may disrupt scrotal thermoregulation and result in derangement in spermatogenesis. Diagnosis is via a combination of digital palpation and ultrasonography. Treatment involves cold water hydrotherapy, NSAIDs, topical antibiotic ointments, systemic antibiotics, cleansing with shampoos, corticosteroids for pruritus, and/or castration with or without scrotal ablation.[57–59] Return to normal spermatogenesis typically occurs 60 to 120 days after resolution of the edema or thickening. If the thickening persists long term, there may be permanent derangement of spermatogenesis.

Fluid Within the Vaginal Space

Fluid within the vaginal space may be a transudate, modified transudate, or exudate and may originate from the abdominal cavity or the scrotum itself.[2,3,27] It may be caused by trauma, inflammation, infection, neoplasia, or foreign body migration and may be unilateral or bilateral. Hematocele (bloody fluid) is typically the result of trauma or vascular disease with capillary rupture. Hydrocele (serous fluid) may be caused by abdominal fluid accumulation (peritonitis, ascites) with leakage through the vaginal rings into the vaginal space, poor lymphatic blood flow associated with scrotal or inguinal herniation, inflammation, parasite migration, or neoplasia.

Signs include malaise, abdominal enlargement, fever, anorexia and scrotal enlargement.[2,3,27] Diagnosis will be made based on physical examination, chemistry and complete blood count, abdominal and/or thoracic radiography, ultrasonography of the abdomen and scrotal contents, and cytology and culture of the fluid. Treatment of

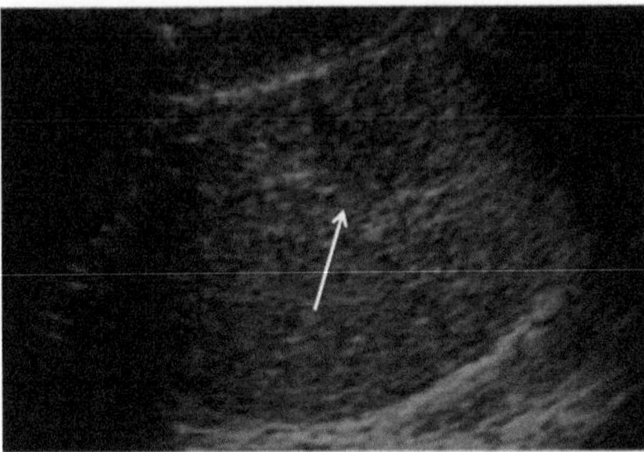

Fig. 6. Testicular seminoma in a dog. A well circumscribed hypoechoic round foci is visible by ultrasound (*arrow*).

the primary disease is indicated plus hemicastration, and systemic antibiotics where indicated. Return to normal spermatogenesis in 90 to 120 days may be expected if the fluid accumulation is not longstanding and completely resolves. Purulent exudate or transudates in the vaginal space may result in adhesion formation, which may affect the ability of the testicle to thermoregulate properly.

Neoplasia

Testicular neoplasia tends to occur in aged male dogs (9–11 years) with an incidence of 1% and is covered in another article by Rob Foster elsewhere in this issue.[2–4,16,24,26] Multiple tumor types may be present in the same testicle. Retained testes or testicles that were retained at some point are at 9 to 11 times greater risk of neoplasia compared to testicles that descended normally. Physical examination may reveal an enlarged testicle(s) or there may be a palpable mass. The surrounding testicular tissue tends to be softer than the tumor. Semen evaluation commonly reveals abnormalities in morphology with primary defects predominating. Ultrasonography may be used to better delineate the tumor(s) (**Fig. 6**). The mediastinum testis may be obliterated or displaced by neoplastic tissue. Testicular aspiration or biopsy may be used to obtain a diagnosis. Histopathology is confirmatory.

In cases where both testicles are affected or the individual is not a breeding male, complete castration is recommended.[2–4,16,24,26] Bilateral castration is recommended for patients with SCT regardless of breeding status because the endocrine secretions from these tumors may have serious health consequences and it is possible that there may be a small metastatic tumor in the opposite testicle that is not visible at the time of initial diagnosis. In a breeding animal, hemicastration may be the preferred method of treatment if the lesion is unilateral. Following hemicastration, if there are no complications, a return to normal spermatogenesis should be expected in 60 to 90 days. Compensatory hypertrophy may occur following hemicastration with two-thirds return to full spermatogenic function possible in some cases within 6 months. Chemotherapy with cisplatin, vinblastine, cyclosphosphamide, and methotrexate is used for metastatic tumors.

The most common types of scrotal neoplasia are squamous cell carcinoma, melanoma, and mast cell tumor,[27] while the most common tumors of the penis and prepuce are squamous cell carcinoma, papilloma, transitional cell carcinoma, mast cell tumors, and transmissible venereal tumors.[2–4,16,24,26,29] Treatment includes surgical excision, cryotherapy, radiation therapy, chemotherapy, or autogenous vaccination protocols.

UNWILLINGNESS/FAILURE TO BREED

Unwillingness or failure to breed may be caused by a variety of causes.[2–4,24] Infection of the prepuce (balanitis), penis (posthitis), prostatitis, or urethritis may result in pain, resulting in unwillingness to breed despite good libido. Initially there may be attempts at breeding followed by unwillingness to mate due to negative reinforcement. Balanoposthitis may be caused by concurrent cystitis, urethritis, or prostatitis, trauma, bacterial sepsis, or lack of mucosal immunity from immunosuppressive conditions. Canine herpesvirus and calicivirus may also be causative. Balanoposthitis may be a component of atopic dermatitis or may be a result of self-mutilation due to anxiety disorders or pruritus. Physical examination may reveal abnormal purulent or bloody preputial discharge, with erosive ulcerative lesions and lymphoid hyperplasia on the penile and preputial mucosa. There may be pain associated with manipulation of the penis either within the preputial sheath or on eversion. Urethritis may present as bloody drippings from the penis, hematuria, or stranguria.

Culture and cytology (touch prep) should be performed and must be differentiated from normal smegma (high numbers of neutrophils, low numbers of rods and cocci, and few intracellular bacteria).[2–4,24] Treatment includes gentle douching of the preputial orifice with water and dilute iodine solution or 1% acetic acid solution. The author recommends treating no more often than every other week. Oral antibiotics based on culture and sensitivity and topical antibiotics may be helpful. Systemic probiotics may help reestablish normal flora. Self-mutilation should be treated with behavior modification or antianxiety medications.

Urethral prolapse typically occurs in younger dogs (9 months–5 years) and the English bulldog is predisposed.[2–4,24] It may be hereditary or may occur secondarily to urethritis or sexual arousal. Usually the entire distal end of the urethra is prolapsed and becomes edematous due to exposure and licking. Clinical signs included intermittent bloody drippings from the prepuce, a doughnut- or pea-shaped pink-red mass of rounded protruding tissue from the end of the penis, and occasionally pollakiuria. Sexual rest and an Elizabethan or neck collar are recommended to prevent self-trauma prior to surgery. Surgery is the treatment of choice and involves replacing and tacking the prolapsed tissue or complete removal of the prolapsed tissue.

Musculoskeletal or neurologic disorders may result in inability to breed due to pain or discomfort during the mating process or weakness.[2–4,24] Hip dysplasia, cruciate injury, spondylosis (thoracic, lumbar, sacral), arthritis, intervertebral disc disease, or muscle wasting due to age or neurologic injury may result in enough pain that breeding is discouraged. Diagnosis and treatment of the primary disorder are paramount. Further treatment is aimed at multimodal pain management. Use of NSAIDs may decrease pain and inflammation. Use of NSAIDs may result in decreased seminal prostaglandin concentrations, which may affect fertility; they may also decrease spermatogenesis and spermiogenesis.[64–66,68] It is best to use them on an as-needed basis in breeding males rather than on a daily basis. Opiate analgesics may be helpful along with NSAID therapy particularly just prior to breeding or collection. If nerve pain is suspected to be a part of the equation, addition of a GABA analogue may be helpful. Nontraditional treatments of acupuncture, chiropractic, and physical therapy all may be beneficial depending on the type of injury present. Manual collection may present an option for those dogs that are still able to ejaculate but simply cannot mount or penetrate due to musculoskeletal disorder.[2–4,24]

Physical detriments including size discrepancy between the male and female, entanglement with hair causing penile injury, laceration and pain, or matted hair over the end of the prepuce or over the vulvar lips may prevent intromission or may result in negative reinforcement for breeding behaviors.[2–4,24] When size is the main discrepancy, manual collection will alleviate this concern. Trimming of long or matted hairs will prevent injury and allow penetration to occur.

Psychological factors are important causes of failure to breed.[2–4,24] Young or inexperienced males are easily discouraged from breeding by dominant females or females that have not reached their receptive period. An aggressive attack by a bitch may scare an insecure male into being unwilling to even attempt a breeding despite normal libido and mating ability. Supervision of breeding will help prevent injuries. Bringing the female to the male's territory or to neutral territory may diminish any protective behaviors that might otherwise be displayed. Breeding experiences should always be positive in order to keep the male willing to attempt breedings with new females.

EJACULATORY DISORDERS

Copulation involves both emission and ejaculation.[3,24,69–71] Emission involves the release of sperm and prostatic fluid from the cauda epididymis, vas deferens, and prostate into the prostatic urethra, followed by closure of the neck of the bladder and propulsion of sperm through the pelvic urethra. It is mediated by sympathetic control via the hypogastric nerve. Ejaculation is the forceful expulsion of these fluids out of the urethra. Rhythmic contractions of the bulbospongiosus, ischiocavernonsus muscles, and other striated pelvic muscles propel sperm and seminal fluid down and out of the penile urethra and via the pudendal nerve to effect ejaculation.

Neurologic injury or dysfunction may result in ejaculatory dysfunction. It may be associated with pelvic injury due to trauma, intervertebral disc disease, cauda equina syndrome, or diabetic polyneuropathy.[3,24,69–71] The primary disease or injury should be treated.

Retrograde ejaculation may result if the sympathetic α-receptors in the bladder neck are blocked due to neurologic dysfunction or medication administration.[3,24,34,35] The result of retrograde ejaculation is a decreased number of sperm in the ejaculate or, in the extreme case, azoospermia. Treatment with α_2-adrenergic agonists, like xylazine or metdetomidine, can cause retrograde ejaculation. Diagnosis is via urine collection by catheterization following semen collection and comparing numbers of sperm in the urine to a normal ejaculate and the ejaculated sample. Treatment involves pretreatment with a sympathomimetic drug like phenylpropanolamine (3 mg/kg orally twice a day or pseudoephedrine (4–5 mg/kg orally 3 times a day or 1 and 3 hours prior to collection or breeding).

Sperm granuloma may result in partial or complete obstruction of one or both epididymides or vas deferens.[2,3,16,17,26,61,62] In azoospermic individuals, it is important to determine if ejaculation has occurred. Presence of high concentrations of alkaline phosphatase concentrations (>5000 IU/L) in the ejaculate provide evidence of ejaculation, while low concentrations (<2500 IU/L) indicate failure to ejaculate, and concentrations between these 2 ranges are equivocal or indicate partial ejaculation.[41] While granulomas are not a cause of ejaculation failure, they may present as failure to ejaculate and are only diagnosed on further examination.

Prepubertal dogs may develop normal erections but fail to ejaculate.[2,3] Other behavioral causes may include fear or intimidation by a dominant female, inexperience, or poor footing resulting in slipping of the hind limbs. Collection in the presence of an estrus teaser may facilitate emission and ejaculation. Treatment with gonadotropin releasing hormone (GnRH), at a dose of 1 to 2 μg/kg SQ or IM, 1 to 3 hours prior to collection may increase libido and the chance that ejaculation will occur.[41] Administration of dinoprost tromethamine (Lutalyse) at a dose of 25 to 100 μg/kg SQ may advance emission and ejaculation without a complete erection or significant libido.[72]

SUMMARY

Infertility in the dog has many potential causes. A careful and systematic approach to diagnosis requires careful history taking, complete physical examination, semen evaluation, and advanced diagnostics including lab work, ultrasonography, and radiography. Once a diagnosis is made, a treatment plan can be formulated. An important part of the treatment plans involves breeding management and requires cooperation from both the dog and bitch owner in order to have successful breeding outcomes.

REFERENCES

1. Lopate C. Advances in canine semen evaluation techniques. Clin Theriogenol 2009; 1:81–90.
2. Meyers-Wallen VN. Clinical approach to infertile male dogs with sperm in the ejaculate. Vet Clin North Am 1991;21:609–33.
3. Johnston SD, Root Kustritz MV, Olson PNS. Clinical approach to infertility in the male dog. In: Canine and feline theriogenology. Philadelphia: WB Saunders; 2001. p. 370–88.
4. Zambelli D, Levy X. Clinical approach to the infertile male. In: BSAVA manual of canine and feline reproduction and neonatology. Cheltenham (UK): British Small Animal Veterinary Association; 2010. p. 70–9.
5. Johnson C. Current concepts on infertility in the dog. Waltham Focus 2006;16:7–12.
6. Johnston SD, Root Kustritz MV, Olson PNS. Semen collection, evaluation, and preservation. In: Canine and feline theriogenology. Philadelphia: WB Saunders; 2001. p. 287–306.
7. Powe JR, Canfield PJ, Martin PA. Evaluation of the cytologic diagnosis of prostatic disorders. Vet Clin Pathol 2004;3:150–4.
8. Root Kustritz MV, Johnston SD, Olson PN, et al. Relationship between inflammatory cytology of canine seminal fluid and significant aerobic bacterial, anaerobic bacterial or Mycoplasma cultures of canine seminal fluid: 95 cases (1987–2000). Theriogenology 2005;64:1333–9.
9. Nunez-Martinez I, Moran JM, Pena FJ. Do computer-assisted morphometric derived sperm characteristics reflect DNA status in canine spermatozoa? Reprod Dom Anim 2005;40:537–43.
10. Johanisson E, Campana A, Luthi R, et al. Evaluation of 'round cells' in semen analysis: a comparative study. Hum Reprod Update 2000;6:404–12.
11. Kumi-Diaka J. Subjecting canine semen to the hypo-osmotic test. Theriogenology 1993;39:1279–89.
12. Pinto CRF, Kozink DM. Simplified hypoosmotic swelling test (HOST) of fresh and frozen-thawed canine spermatozoa. Anim Reprod Sci 2008;104:450–5.
13. Peña AI, Quintela LA, Herradón PG. Viability assessment of dog spermatozoa using flow cytometry. Theriogenology 1998;50:1211–20.
14. Peña AI, Quintela LA, Heradon PG. Flow cytometric assessment of acrosomal status and viability of dog spermatozoa. Reprod Dom Anim 1999;34:495–502.
15. Everson DP, Wixon R. Clinical aspects of sperm DNA fragmentation detection and male infertility. Theriogenology 2006;65:979–91.

16. Olson PN. Clinical approach for evaluating dogs with azoospermia or aspermia. Vet Clin North Am 1991;21:591–608.
17. Olson PN, Schultheiss P, Seim HB. Clinical and laboratory findings associated with actual or suspected azoospermia in dogs: 18 cases (1979–1990). J Am Vet Med Assoc 1992;201:478–82.
18. Metcalfe SS, Gunn IM, Champness KA. Azoospermia in two Labrador retrievers. Aust Vet J 1999;77:570–3.
19. Kawakami E, Amemiya E, Namikawa K, et al. High plasma estradiol-17β levels in dogs with benign prostatic hyperplasia and azoospermia. J Vet Med Sci 2001;63:407–12.
20. Kipperman BS, Wong VJ, Plopper CG. Primary ciliary dyskinesia in a Gordon setter. J Am Anim Hosp Assoc 1992;28:375–9.
21. Edwards DF, Patton DS, Bemis DA, et al. Immotile cilia syndrome in three dogs from a litter. J Am Vet Med Assoc 1983;183:667–72.
22. Vaden LS, Breitschwerdt EB, Henrikson, CK, et al. Primary ciliary dyskinesia in Bichon Frise litter mates. J Am Anim Hosp Assoc 1991;27:633–40.
23. Randolph JF, Castleman WL. Immotile cilia syndrome in two olde English sheepdog litter-mates. J Small Anim Pract 1984;25:679–86.
24. Lopate C. Clinical approach to conditions of the male. In: Manual of canine and feline reproduction and neonatology. Gloucester (UK): British Small Animal Veterinary Association; 2010. p. 191–211.
25. Kukk A. Emerging roles for vitamin D and prolactin in canine male reproduction. Clin Theriogenol 2011;3:226–32.
26. Johnston SD, Root Kustritz MV, Olson PNS. Disorders of the canine testes and epididymes. In: Canine and feline theriogenology. Philadelphia: WB Saunders; 2001. p. 312–32.
27. Johnston SD, Root Kustritz MV, Olson PNS. Disorders of the canine scrotum. In: Canine and feline theriogenology. Philadelphia: WB Saunders; 2001. p. 333–6.
28. Johnston SD, Root Kustritz MV, Olson PNS. Disorders of the canine prostate. In: Canine and feline theriogenology. Philadelphia: WB Saunders; 2001. p. 337–55.
29. Johnston SD, Root Kustritz MV, Olson PNS. Disorders of the canine penis and prepuce. In: Canine and feline theriogenology. Philadelphia: WB Saunders; 2001. p. 356–67.
30. Dorfman M, Barsanti J. Diseases of the canine prostate gland. Compendium 1995; 17:791–806.
31. Froman DP, Amann RP. Inhibition of motility of bovine, canine and equine spermatozoa by artificial vaginal lubricants. Theriogenology 1983;20:357–61.
32. Fritz TE, Lombard LS, Tyler SA. Pathology and familial incidence of orchitis and its relation to thyroiditis in a closed beagle colony. Exp Mol Pathol 1976;24:142–58.
33. Allen WE, Patel JR. Autoimmune orchitis in two related dogs. J Small Anim Pract 1982;23:713–8.
34. Root MV, Johnston SD, Olson PN. Concurrent retrograde ejaculation and hypothyroidism in a dog: a case report. Theriogenology 1994;41:593–600.
35. Beaufays F, Onclin K, Verstegen J. Retrograde ejaculation occurs in the dog, but can be prevented by pre-treatment with phenylpropanolamine: a urodynamic study. Theriogenology 2008;70:1057–64.
36. Taylor RM, Martin ICA, Faroow BRH. Reproduction abnormalities in canine fucosidosis. J Comp Pathol 1989;100:369–80.
37. Romagnoli S, Bonaccini P, Stellatta C, et al. Clinical use of testicular fine needle aspiration cytology in oligospermic and azoospermic dogs. Reprod Dom Anim 2009;44(Suppl 2):329–33.

38. Dahlbom M, Mäkinen A, Suominen J. Testicular fine needle aspiration cytology as a diagnostic tool in dog infertility. J Sm Anim Pract 1997;38:506–12.
39. Santos M, Marcos R, Caniatti M. Cytologic study of the normal canine testis. Theriogenology 2010;73:208–14.
40. Lopate C, Threlfall WR, Rosol TJ. Histopathologic and gross effects of testicular biopsy in the dog. Therio 1989;32:585–602.
41. Frenette G, Dubé, Tremblay RR. Origin of alkaline phosphatase of canine seminal plasma. Arch Androl 1986;16:235–41.
42. Kawakami E, Masaoaka Y, Hirano T, et al. Changes in plasma testosterone levels and semen quality after 3 injections of a GnRH analogue in 3 dogs with spermatogenic dysfunction. J Vet Med Sci 2005;67:1249–52.
43. Loza ME, Wanke MM, Monachesi NE, et al. Effects of human chorionic gonadotrophin (HCG) on dog semen quality. Proceedings of the 6th International Symposium on Canine and Feline Reproduction. Vienna (Austria); 2008. p. 139.
44. Kawakami E, Hori T, Tsutsui T. Changes in plasma LH and testosterone levels and semen quality after a single injection of hCG in 2 dogs with spermatogenic dysfunction. J Vet Med Sci 1998;60:765–7.
45. Kawakami E, Hori T, Tsutsui T. Changes in plasma luteinizing hormone, testosterone and estradiol 17β levels and semen quality after injections of gonadotropin releasing hormone agonist and human chorionic gonadotropin in three dogs with oligozoospermia and two dogs with azoospermia. Anin Reprod Sci 1997;47:157–67.
46. Kawakami E, Hori T, Tsutsui T. Changes in plasma testosterone and testicular transferrin concentration, testicular histology and semen quality after treatment of testosterone-depot plus PMSG to 3 dogs with asthenozoospermia. J Vet Med Sci 2000;62:203–6.
47. Kawakami E, Tonsho H, Tsutsui T, et al. Effects of LHRH-analogue treatment of spermatogenic dysfunction in the dog. Int J Androl 1991;14:441–52.
48. Kawakami E, Taguchi N, Hirano T, et al. Therapeutic effect of aromatase inhibitor in two azoospermic dogs with high plasma estradiol 17β levels. J Vet Med Sci 2003; 65:1343–5.
49. Bjurström L, Linde-Forsberg C. Long-term study of aerobic bacteria of the genital tract in stud dogs. Am J Vet Res 1992;53;670–3.
50. Kamolpatana K, Johnston SD, Hardy SK, et al. Effect of finasteride on serum concentration of dihydrotestosterone and testosterone in three clinically normal sexually intact adult male dogs. Am J Vet Res 1998;59:762–4.
51. Iguer-Ouada M, Verstegen JP. Effect of finasteride (Proscar MSD) on seminal composition, prostate function and fertility in male dogs. J Reprod Fertil Suppl 1997;51: 139–9.
52. Sirinarumitr K, Johnston SD, Root Kustritz MV, et al. Effects of finasteride on size of the prostate gland and semen quality in dogs with benign prostatic hypertrophy. J Am Vet Med Assoc 2001;218:1275–80.
53. Albouy M, Sanquer A, Maynard L. Efficacies of osaterone and delmadinone in the treatment of benign prostatic hyperplasia in dogs. Vet Rec 2008;163:179–83.
54. Tsutsui T, Hori T, Shimizu M, et al. Regression of prostate hypertrophy by osaterone acetate in dogs. J Vet Med Sci 2000;62:1115–9.
55. Tsutsui T, Hori T, Shimizu M, et al. Effect of osaterone acetate administration on prostatic regression rate, peripheral bloody hormone levels and semen quality in dogs with benign prostatic hypertrophy. J Vet Med Sci 2001;63:453–6.
56. Gonzalez G, Guendualain C, Maffrand C. Comparison of the effect of the aromatase inhibitor, anastrazole, to the antioestrogen, tamoxifen citrate on canine prostate and semen. Reprod Dom Anim 2009;44(Suppl 2):316–9.

57. Glynn MK, Lynn TV. Brucellosis. J Am Vet Med Assoc 2008;233;900–8.
58. Wanke MM. Canine brucellosis. Anim Reprod Sci 2004;82–83:195–207.
59. Hollett B. Canine brucellosis: outbreaks and compliance. Therio 2006;66:575–87.
60. Dorfman M, Barsanti J, Budsberg SC. Enrofloxacin concentrations in dogs with normal prostate and dogs with chronic bacterial prostatitis. Am J Vet Res 1995;56: 386–90.
61. Foley GL, Bassily N, Hess RA. Intratubular spermatic granulomas of the canine efferent ductules. Toxicol Pathol 1995;23:731–4.
62. Kawakami E, Koga H, Hori T, et al. Sperm granuloma and sperm agglutination in a dog with asthenozoospermia. J Vet Med Sci 2003;65:409–12.
63. Moskovitz B, Munichor M, Levin DR. Effect of diclofenac sodium (Voltaren) and prostaglandin E2 on spermatogenesis in mature dogs. Eur Urol 1987;13:393–6.
64. Didolkar AK, Patel PB, Roychowdhury D. Effect of aspirin on spermatogenesis in mature and immature rats. Int J Androl 1980;3:585–93.
65. Winnall WR, Muir JA, Liew S, et al. Effects of chronic celecoxib on testicular function in normal and lipopolysaccharide-treated rats. Int J Androl 2009;32:542–55.
66. Wiger R, Hongslo JK, Evenson DP, et al. Effects of acetaminophen and hydroxyurea on spermatogenesis and sperm chromatin structure in laboratory mice. Reprod Toxicol 1995;9:21–33.
67. Purswell BJ, Wilcke JR. Response to GnRH by the intact male dog: testosterone, LH, and FSH levels. J Reprod Fertil Suppl 1993;47:335–41.
68. Allen WE, Longstaffe JA. Spermatogenic arrest associated with focal degenerative orchitis in related dogs. J Small Anim Pract 1982;23:337–43.
69. McDonnell SM. Ejaculation: physiology and dysfunction. Vet Clin North Am Equine 1992;8:57–70.
70. Thomas AJ. Ejaculatory dysfunction. Fertil Steril 1989;39:445–54.
71. Arver S, Sjöstrand NO. Function of adrenergic and cholinergic nerves in canine effectors of seminal emission. Acta Physiol Scand 1982;115:67–77.
72. Kustritz MV, Hess M. Effect of administration of prostaglandin F2alpha or presence of an estrous teaser bitch on characteristics of the canine ejaculate. Theriogenology 2007;67:255–8.

Guide to Emergency Interception During Parturition in the Dog and Cat

Frances O. Smith, DVM, PhD[a,b,*]

KEYWORDS

• Parturition • Emergency • Bitch • Queen

Parturition in the dog and cat allows many opportunities for emergency intervention to become necessary. Knowledge of normal parturition is a requirement for the emergency situation to be properly identified. Clients who are breeders of purebred dogs and cats may be able to alert the attending clinician to observed problems with a particular parturition, but many of the emergency presentation will involve owners with little background information on the bitch or queen and inaccurate information related to breeding dates or even when the breeding did occur.

Normal gestation in the bitch is approximately 63 days with a range of 56 to 72 days from date of first known breeding. The variability in gestation length is due to the long life span of the spermatozoa in the genital tract of the bitch. When calculated from the date of the luteinizing hormone peak or from the date of ovulation, gestation is much more predictable with a gestation length of 65 ± 1 day from the luteinizing hormone surge or 63 ± 1 day from ovulation.[1,2] Litter size can have an effect on gestation length, with gestation being shorter for large litters and longer for smaller litters.

Normal gestation in the queen is approximately 65 days with a range of 52 to 74 days from breeding to the onset of parturition.[3,4] The queen is an induced ovulator and may allow multiple matings to the same or multiple toms over a period of several days. A queen that is bred by more than 1 male may have kittens sired by different toms (superfecundation). A cat breeder will often have breeding dates recorded, but the accidently bred or casually bred queen will typically present with no information on breeding dates. Length of gestation in the queen is influenced both by litter size and by breed, although litter size is not as well correlated with gestation length in the

The author has nothing to disclose.

[a] Orthopedic Foundation for Animals, Inc, 2300 East Nifong Boulevard, Columbia, MO 65201, USA
[b] Smith Veterinary Hospital, 1110 Highway 13 East, Burnsville, MN 55337, USA
* Smith Veterinary Hospital, 1110 Highway 13 East, Burnsville, MN 55337.
E-mail address: zacrescendo@comcast.net

Vet Clin Small Anim 42 (2012) 489–499
doi:10.1016/j.cvsm.2012.02.001 **vetsmall.theclinics.com**
0195-5616/12/$ – see front matter

Box 1
Breeds of dog with high incidence of dystocia

- Boston Terrier
- Scottish Terrier
- Pekinese
- Mastiff
- Clumber Spaniel
- Dandie Dinmont
- French Bulldog
- German Wirehair Pointer
- Bulldog
- Miniature Bulldog

queen as it is in the bitch.[4] The Burmese breed is reported to have an average litter size of 5 kittens, and the chinchilla cat, an average litter size of 2.8 kittens.[5]

There are 3 stages of parturition in both the bitch and the queen. Stage I is clinically unapparent and is marked by increasing uterine contraction and gradual cervical dilation. Stage I labor in the bitch typically lasts 6 to 12 hours but may last as long as 36 hours. A bitch can delay parturition when she is nervous or in unfamiliar and busy surroundings. During this period the bitch is typically restless, pants, may refuse food, and begins nesting behavior. Duration of stage I labor in the queen may be shorter and is characterized by vocalization, rapid breathing, restlessness, and loud purring. Stage II involves the process of fetal expulsion through the fully dilated cervix. This stage typically lasts 3 to 12 hours in the bitch (averaging about 1 puppy per hour) and 4 to 16 hours in the queen with an occasional queen delivering the last kitten after 42 hours. Parturition length of beyond 42 hours is not normal. Stage III labor involves placental passage. A placenta typically follows delivery of the fetus either immediately or within 15 minutes. Several placentas may be delivered at once.

Dystocia or difficult birth is the most commonly encountered emergency occurring during parturition. Rate of dystocia varies from 2% (of insured dogs in Sweden) to an overall reported dystocia rate of 5%.[6] In the queen, the incidence of dystocia is reported as 3.3% to 5.8% of parturitions.[7] Risk factors for dystocia include breed, age of bitch, parity, litter size, and body size of bitch. Older primiparous bitches (>6 years of age) have a significantly increased risk of having problems during parturition and have an increased incidence of stillbirths. Breeds with a high incidence of dystocia are provided in **Box 1.** Bitches of miniature and small breeds had an increased incidence of dystocia.[8] Uterine inertia and spasm, malpresentation of the fetus, and single pup or large litter size are the most common causes for dystocia. Breeds with the highest caesarean rates are brachycephalic breeds, terrier breeds, Pekinese and a few gundogs.[8] In the Boston terrier, bulldog, and French bulldog, the cesarean rate is greater than 80%.[8]

A summary for the clinical signs associated with dystocia is provided in **Box 2**. Clinical signs associated with a diagnosis of dystocia are failure to deliver a fetus for longer than 24 hours after the onset of stage I labor, a temperature drop below 99°F (30°C), 60 minutes of active labor with no fetus delivered, protrusion of fetal membranes from the vulva for 15 minutes or longer without delivery of the fetus,

Box 2
Criteria for diagnosis of dystocia in the dog and cat

- Prolonged gestation when ovulation is known
- Pregnant bitch >72 days post breeding
- Pregnant queen >71 days post breeding
- Bitch strains for 1 hour continuously before the delivery of any puppy
- Green or black vaginal discharge prior to delivery of first puppy
- The bitch rests 3 or more hours between puppies
- The delivery of stillborn puppies
- The dam is ill or distressed

greater than 3 hours since delivery of last fetus when more fetuses are present, presence of greenish-black discharge prior to delivery of the first fetus, signs of weakness or illness in the dam, and/or vaginal hemorrhage during labor. Dystocia should also be considered if the bitch has gone greater than 70 days since the first breeding or 71 days in the queen.[9]

Dystocia can be caused by maternal factors (including primary or secondary uterine inertia, pelvic fracture, uterine torsion, vaginal abnormalities such as bands, malnutrition, and parasitism) or by fetal causes.[10] Fetal causes include fetal monster, anasarcous fetuses, cephalopelvic disproportion, true fetal oversize or disproportion between fetal size and dam size, and fetal death. In the bitch, 75.3% of the dystocias have been classified as maternal in origin with 24.7% classified as fetal in origin.[11] In the queen, 67.1% of the dystocias are maternal in origin and 29.7% are fetal in origin. Primary and secondary uterine inertia are the most common cause for dystocia of maternal origin.[12,13] Malpresentation of the fetus is the most common cause of dystocia of fetal origin.

The normal position of the fetus is anterior or posterior presentation (relates long axis of the fetus to that of the bitch), dorsal position (which surface of the uterus the fetal vertebral column is in contact with), and fully extended posture (refers to the location of the head and extremities of the fetus) (**Fig. 1**). Posterior presentation with rear limbs extended is normal in the dog and cat; however, a true breech in which the hips are flexed under the fetus is not normal and can result in dystocia. Approximately 70% of kittens have an anterior presentation: 60% to 70% of puppies have an anterior presentation. Posterior presentations are considered normal in both the bitch and the queen but do present an increased risk for neonatal mortality. Transverse presentation can occur and are responsible for a substantial percentage of dystocias of fetal origin. With transverse presentation, the bitch may stop uterine contractions. Occasionally, 2 fetuses may attempt to enter the uterine body at the same time resulting in a "traffic" jam. Many cases of dystocia are associated with fetal malposition.[13]

Primary and secondary uterine inertia are the most common causes of dystocia of maternal origin.[14–16] Primary uterine inertia may be either complete or partial—primary uterine inertia is a failure of the uterus to contract or to contract in an organized fashion.[12] A bitch or queen with complete primary uterine inertia does not reach stage II of labor. A bitch or queen with partial primary inertia reaches stage II of labor but attempts to deliver the fetus are weak and unsuccessful. Secondary uterine inertia can occur from both anatomic and physiologic causes. Persistent uterine contractions

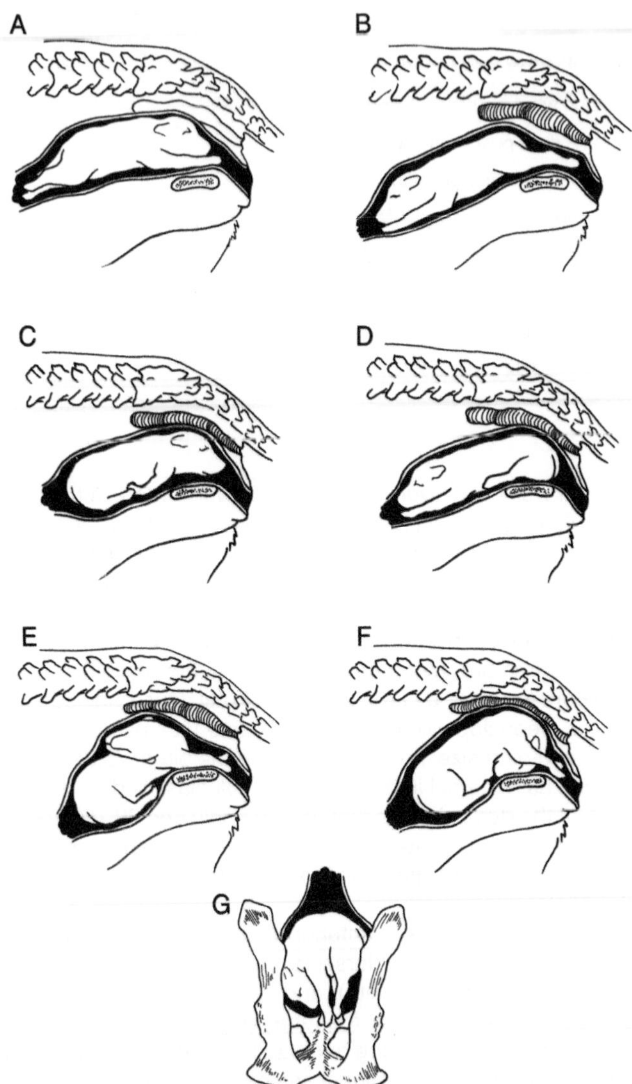

Fig. 1. Fetal presentation and postures. (*From* Johnston SD, Olsen PNS, Root Kustritz MV. Canine and feline theriogenology. Philadelphia: WB Saunders; 2001; with permission.)

against an obstructed birth canal (ie, transverse presentation) or delivery of a large litter can result in exhaustion of the uterine musculature.

Uterine torsion is an important differential as a cause of secondary uterine inertia. Uterine torsion has been reported in both the bitch and the queen. The bitch or queen may be very depressed and have injected sclera, tachycardia, and slow capillary refill time. The abdomen is often very painful. Uterine torsion is diagnosed more frequently in the queen than in the bitch and may occur at term or prior to term.[16,17] It is important to assess the underlying cause of the dystocia before selecting a treatment regimen.

DIAGNOSIS OF DYSTOCIA

A complete physical examination should be performed to assess temperature, pulse, respiration, hydration status, and capillary refill time to assess overall maternal health. Check the sclera for injection, which indicates stress. Auscultate the chest, examine the abdomen, and perform a vaginal examination on the bitch to identify a fetus in the vagina. Confirm that the bitch or queen is pregnant—cat breeders may over interpret changes in the queen as confirmation of pregnancy. When in doubt, an abdominal radiograph is warranted and will allow the assessment of litter size. The bitch or queen should have a complete blood count and serum chemistries, including calcium and glucose, performed.

It is important to keep the owner informed of the diagnosis, prognosis for survival of the dam and offspring, and the expected costs involved with all procedures. This author recommends that any client considering a breeding carefully evaluate the financial, personal, and ethical requirements necessary to produce healthy offspring. This author recommends that the client be prepared to sustain a financial loss of several thousand dollars. Many cases of dystocia can be managed medically but 60% to 80% of the dystocias treated require surgical intervention. The client should be informed that fetal death in both species rises rapidly with prolonged stage II labor. In bitches, fetal deaths increase from 5.8% in labors of 1 to 4.5 hours to 13.7% in bitches treated 5 to 24 hours after onset of stage II labor.[11] Cesarean section should not be a last resort as puppy survivability is an important consideration in the management of dystocia.[17] Ultrasonography, if available, is the ideal method to assess fetal stress and viability. The normal canine fetal heart rate is greater than 200 beats/min. Normal fetal heart rate in the cat averages 228.2 $\pm$ 35.5 beats/min. A fetal heart rate less than 180 beats/min is a sign of fetal distress, whereas a fetal heart rate less than 160 beats/min warrants emergency intervention. The fetal heart rate slows with hypoxia, unlike the adult animal. Rapid intervention during dystocia can reduce fetal mortality from 9% to 3%.[16,17]

MEDICAL MANAGEMENT OF DYSTOCIA

Medical management for relief of dystocia is indicated when the dam is healthy, the labor has not been too long, the cervix is confirmed to be dilated either by visual examination of the cervix or by prior delivery of a fetus, fetal size is appropriate for vaginal delivery, and the fetal heart rate is normal or near normal.[14] Medical management may also be indicated when there is only one remaining fetus after an otherwise unremarkable parturition or when it is certain that the remaining fetus is dead. Medical management cannot be used in cases of obstructive dystocia whether due to maternal or fetal causes. Medical management may also be unsuccessful if multiple fetuses remain in utero due to maternal and/or uterine fatigue.

Medical management of dystocia typically involves the use of the ecbolic drug oxytocin and/or calcium gluconate and glucose. Oxytocin is a hormone produced by neurons in the hypothalamus. During pregnancy, the myometrium is particularly sensitive to oxytocin, and a rise in plasma oxytocin coincides with the first labor contraction. Oxytocin has historically been administered at many different doses ranging from 5 to 20 U IM in the dog and 2 to 4 U IM in the cat. Currently recommended doses are 0.5 to 2 U to increase the frequency and quality of uterine contractions. Initial doses of 0.1 U/kg are recommended. The dosage may be repeated in 30 minutes. This author never administers more than 2 doses of oxytocin due to the risk of uterine hyperstimulation and fetal distress associated with placental separation.[18]

Calcium is often used in addition to oxytocin or may be used when concentration of total or ionized calcium are known to be low. Calcium ions are necessary for myometrial contraction. Calcium gluconate is available as several salts and is administered as 10% calcium gluconate at 0.2 mL/kg IV or 1 to 5 mL per dog SC. Cardiac arrhythmias are a potential complication when the drug is administered IV, so the chest should be ausculted for any arrhythmias prior to administration. In the queen, calcium use is controversial, due to the very strong uterine contractions seen when it is administered. ECBOLIC DRUGS ARE ABSOLUTELY CONTRAINDICATED IN CASES OF OBSTRUCTIVE DYSTOCIA.[16]

MECHANICAL INTERVENTIONS WITH DYSTOCIA

Manual correction of dystocia by manipulation of the fetus in the bitch or queen can be successful provided the fetus is of normal size. A malpresentation or malposition can sometimes be corrected by a combination of generous use of sterile lubricants and careful manipulation of the fetus. The posture and presentation of the fetus may be assessed by digital examination of the vaginal vault. Instruments such as spay hooks, sponge forceps, and clamshell forceps can be used but must be applied very carefully as there is very little room for these instruments within the already crowded vaginal vault. Improper application can result in significant soft tissue trauma to the vulva and vagina. Excessive pressure applied with the forceps to the head or jaws of the fetus can results in a fractured or dismembered jaw or a crushed skull. The safest instrument for the extraction of the fetus is the fingers. It is best to grasp the fetus with a gauze or cloth sponge and gently twist and/or lift the fetus up and over the ischial arch (posterior and then ventral direction). The traction should be applied in concert with straining by the dam. In many cases, application of a towel to the caudal abdomen of the bitch in a slinglike fashion can help to push a fetus far enough caudally that it can be grasped and delivered per vagina. If traction and manipulation are not successful within a short period of time, it is prudent to proceed to surgical intervention. If a single fetus is stuck in the vaginal vault that cannot be extracted using lubrication and manipulation, an episiotomy can be considered. Episiotomy can be performed under local, epidural or general anesthesia.

Episiotomy is best performed in a standing position and requires identification and protection of the urethra prior to incision. After delivery of the fetus, the episiotomy is closed in three layers. Technique for episiotomy will not be described here but can be found in any standard surgery text. After an episiotomy, the bitch or queen may be at increased risk for dystocia as a result of scarring secondary to the previous procedure.

SURGICAL TREATMENT OF DYSTOCIA

Failure of manipulative or medical management of dystocia is common. Greater than 60% of the dystocias in bitches and queens result in surgical intervention. Cesarean section is commonly performed in small animal practices, especially practices with populations owning valuable bitches and queens and in emergency and critical care facilities. A large percentage of cesarean sections are performed on an emergency basis. Studies in both the human and small animal population show low risk and good outcomes for planned cesarean section but greatly increase risk to both the mother and the offspring when cesarean section must be performed on an emergency basis.[17]

Determination of the need for emergency cesarean section is based on the assessment of the dam, the progression of the labor, and fetal heart rate.[16] Rapid intervention is the key to survival of the offspring so delays in decision-making and selection of protocol should be minimized. A reduction in fetal heart rate is one of the prime indicators of the need for an emergency cesarean. Ultrasonographic detection of fetal heart rates less than 150 beats/min in 1 or more fetuses indicates severe fetal stress, and cesarean section should be performed immediately to maximize fetal survival. A heart rate in the fetus of 150 to 170 indicates moderate to severe stress and cesarean section should be considered. The heart rate of a fetus should be confirmed with multiple readings over several minutes (2 to 3) to be certain that a drop in heart rate is not occurring coincident with a uterine contraction. Other indications for surgical intervention in dystocia include primary uterine inertia, secondary uterine inertia, obstructive dystocia, and suspicion of uterine rupture or uterine torsion.

The client should be educated on the pros and cons of cesarean section. No surgery is without risk, and the client should be told that the longer the dystocia is allowed to continue, the greater is the risk to both the dam and the neonates. While there are many protocols published regarding cesarean section, it is vital to stabilize the dam with intravenous fluids as needed. Any metabolic abnormalities detected should be managed as rapidly as possible to minimize further compromise to the fetuses. This author does not perform ovariohysterectomy at the time of cesarean section, unless there is irreparable damage to the uterus or ovary. Ovariohysterectomy at the time of cesarean section does increase the risk of hemorrhage and hypovolemic shock due to the large fluid volume associated with the gravid uterus. If an ovariohysterectomy is necessary, the dam will lactate normally provided her nutritional and fluid needs are met and her pain is well controlled. A bitch or queen that undergoes a cesarean section can deliver vaginally at future pregnancies provided that the cause for the dystocia does not recur. The uterus heals very rapidly and the bitch may be bred at her next cycle without an increased risk for uterine rupture. There is no magic number of cesarean sections that bitch or queen can undergo.

Anesthetic protocols should be based on minimizing the time from induction to delivery of all neonates, maintenance of maternal airway, maternal blood pressure, and support of uterine blood flow and should have minimal negative effect on fetal survival. Fetal hypoxia and depression lead to increased fetal loss. It is the author's opinion that all bitches and queens undergoing cesarean section must be intubated to prevent aspiration and to maintain appropriate oxygenation. Many reports have been published recommending and discouraging particular drugs or drugs during cesarean section. The clinician should apply the technique that is most familiar and successful for him or her. No one protocol is ideal; however, xylazine, metdetomidine, ketamine, thiopental, thiamylal, and methoxyflurane are best avoided.[19]

Anticholinergic drugs decrease salivation and prevent excess vagal tone during uterine traction. Fetal cardiac output is dependent on fetal heart rate, not blood pressure, so it is necessary to prevent fetal bradycardia by the administration of an anticholinergic. Opioids have several advantages including excellent pain control and reversibility. Short-acting opioids are preferred so that the duration of action does not exceed the duration of action of the reversal agent. Many protocols suggest the use of propofol for induction. Propofol can cause respiratory depression and apnea when given rapidly IV. Propofol does cross the placental barrier and is found in the umbilical vein of human babies at 13% of the concentration found in maternal blood.[20] Gas anesthetics all cross the placental barrier and will reach the fetus, so exposure time to inhalants should be minimized. Isoflurane and sevoflurane are preferred over halothane for cesarean section. For the dam, remember to prevent bradycardia (treat with atropine) and to prevent tachycardia (treat pain with opioid analgesic), maintain anesthetic depth, and monitor blood pressure.

The dam's blood pressure should be monitored and maintained above 60 mm Hg. If the dam becomes hypotensive, decrease anesthetic concentration, administer an IV fluid bolus, and ensure that blood loss is not excessive. Blood loss during surgery should be replaced at a level of 3 mL of crystalloid for every 1 mL of blood lost. Local blocks are often used to minimize postoperative pain and to supplement general anesthesia. Epidural anesthesia is preferred by some practitioners but has the disadvantage of inability to intubate and oxygenate the bitch and excitability of the bitch when she is positioned for surgery and hears the newborns vocalize.

Either a ventral midline or flank approach to the abdomen may be performed.[20] For the standard ventral approach, a midline incision is made from cranial to the umbilicus to just above the pubis. A very large litter may require an even larger incision. The uterine horns should be exteriorized and packed off using laparotomy sponges. A single uterine body incision should be made if possible. With a very large litter or in cases of uterine torsion or compromise, more than one incision may be necessary to facilitate speed of delivery. Each individual fetus is milked toward the incision site or sites to facilitate delivery. The uterus should be carefully examined from each ovary to the pelvic canal to be sure that all fetuses are completely removed. Removal of each placenta is optional if the cervix is open as spontaneous delivery of the placentas will occur. If the placentas are firmly attached, it is best to allow them to pass without traction as increased uterine hemorrhage can occur with forceful removal. The uterine incision or incisions are closed in 2 layers of an absorbable suture in an inverting pattern. Oxytocin administration of 0.25 to 2.0 IU into the uterine wall will facilitate involution and the passage of any remaining placentas. Following closure of the uterus, lavage the abdomen with sterile warmed fluids and remove any debris or excess. The abdomen may be infused with ampicillin sodium if there is a possibility of contamination. The abdomen is closed in 3 or 4 layers with the linea closed with either nonabsorbable monofilament or polydioxanone suture. The subcutaneous and subcuticular closure is routine. The skin may be closed with either suture or staples.

For a flank incision, the dam is positioned in lateral recumbency and an incision is made behind the last rib extending from just below the epaxial muscles to just above the mammary gland. The skin, subcutaneous tissue, and outer abdominal muscle are incised. Using blunt dissection, the external and internal abdominal obliques are split along the direction of the muscle fibers. The uterine horns are lifted and incised at an appropriate location. The fetuses are again milked toward the uterine incisions for delivery either with or without the placenta that is attached to each fetus. Lateral recumbency allows the dam to breathe more effectively due to decrease pressure on her diaphragm. The major disadvantage of this technique is the longer surgical time as most practitioners in the United States will be inexperienced in this procedure.

An alternative technique for delivery of the litter is an en bloc surgery. In this technique, the ovarian and uterine arteries are clamped or ligated and the entire uterus is removed and handed en bloc to waiting assistants. The assistant opens the uterus and begins immediate resuscitation of the litter. This technique can result in decreased neonatal survival if resuscitation is not prompt and effective. The time from when the first clamp of the arteries to when all neonates have been delivered should be less than 60 seconds. One published study concluded that the outcome was equal to a standard caesarean section result, but the study did not include a control group.[20] The en bloc technique is suitable when the litter is known to be dead and the client does not desire future litters from this dam.

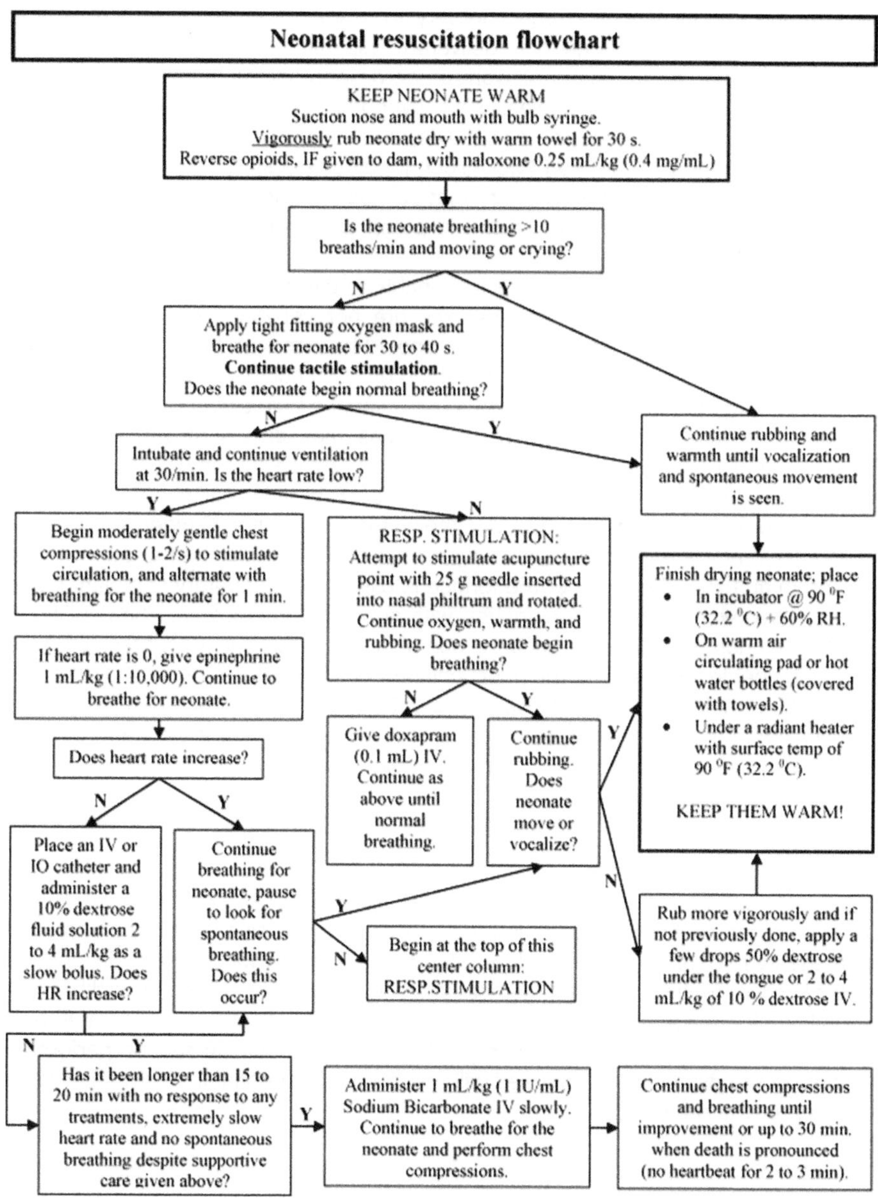

Fig. 2. Flowchart summarizing resuscitation strategy of canine and feline neonates. (*From* Traas AM. Resuscitation of canine and feline neonates. Theriogenology 2008;70:343–8; with permission.)

Resuscitation of the neonates requires trained assistants.[21] There are 2 causes of fetal depression associated with cesarean section: the first is the hypoxia associated with dystocia and the second is depression from medications given to the dam as part of the anesthetic protocol. The neonate responds to hypoxia with slowing of the heart rate, respiratory rate, and movements. Rescuscitation should center on warming the neonate and supplementing oxygen delivery to tissues. For optimal outcome, it is ideal to have 1 assistant per neonate delivered. This may not always be possible in a clinic environment. An incubator or warmer, an oxygen source, a hair dryer, towels, bulb syringes, small-gauge needles, 1-mL syringes, naloxone, epinephrine, doxapram, monitoring equipment, isotonic fluids, and dextrose are all necessary supplies.[20] A new product, One Puff (McCulloch Medical, Auckland, New Zealand), is a simple aspiration/resuscitation product that can be used in any small neonate. It is designed to clear the respiratory tract and pump air into the mask, stimulating the respiratory reflex (**Fig. 2**).

The neonate must be kept warm as it is unable to thermoregulate at birth because the shivering and vasoconstriction reflexes are not yet developed. As soon the neonate is delivered, the fetal membranes should be removed from the head and it should be rubbed dry with a towel. The rubbing often stimulates respiration. The nose and mouth should be cleared of all debris using either a bulb syringe or the One Puff. Stimulation of the umbilical and genital regions may also stimulate respiration. Rubbing the hair backward, performing a gentle accordion motion will also stimulate respiration. Normal newborn respiration is 10 to 18 breaths per minute. Once the neonate is breathing, it may be placed in the warmed incubator. Oxygen supplementation is helpful if a revived neonate remains cyanotic for more than a few minutes. Doxapram at 1 to 2 drops under the tongue is used as a respiratory stimulant but is only effective when used in conjunction with supplemental oxygen. The JenChung GV26 acupuncture has been used to stimulate respiration in neonates. Using a 25-gauge needle inserted into the nasal philtrum until it contacts bone, the needle is whirled to stimulate respiration. Neonates with persistently slow heart rates may benefit from lateral chest compressions to stimulate heart rate. If the dam received narcotics as part of the anesthetic regimen, naloxone at a dose of 0.002 to 0.02 mg/kg IV may be given after delivery.

SUMMARY

Rapid intervention in bitches and queens presenting with dystocia can result in a better outcome for both the dam and the neonates. A decisive diagnostic approach is necessary to determine if dystocia is occurring, the cause for the dystocia, and the most effective treatment option. Medical intervention is often attempted with unsuccessful results. Medical intervention is most likely to be effective in moderate-sized litters when the dam has partial primary uterine inertia. Cesarean section performed as soon as the dystocia is diagnosed will result in higher neonatal survival and rapid recovery for the dam.

REFERENCES

1. Johnston SD, Olsen PNS, Root Kustritz MV. Canine parturition: eutocia and dystocia. In: Canine and feline theriogenology. Philadelphia: WB Saunders; 2001. p. 105–28.
2. Davidson A. Problems during and after parturition. In: Canine and feline reproduction and neonatology. 2nd edition. Quedgeley (UK): BSAVA; 2010. p. 121–34.
3. Root Kustritz MV. Clinical management of pregnancy in cats. Theriogenology 2006; 66:145–50.
4. Johnston SD, Olsen PNS, Root Kustritz MV. Feline parturition. In: Canine and feline theriogenology. Philadelphia: WB Saunders; 2001. p. 431–7.
5. Johnston SD, Olsen PNS, Root Kustritz MV. Feline pregnancy. In: Canine and feline theriogenology. Philadelphia: WB Saunders; 2001. p. 414.

6. Bergstrom A, Egenvall A, Lagerstedt A, et al. Incidence and breed predilection for dystocia and risk factors for cesarean section in a Swedish population of insured dogs. Vet Surg 2006;35:786–91.
7. Ekstrand C, Linde-Forsberg C. Dystocia in the cat: a retrospective study of 155 cases. J Sm Anim Pract 2008;35:459–64.
8. Kuchenmeister U, Munnich A. Dystocia in numbers: evidence-based parameters for intervention in the dog: causes for dystocia and treatment recommendations. Reprod Domest Anim 2009;44:141–7.
9. Adams VJ, Evans KM. Proportion of litters of purebred dogs born by caesarean section. J Sm Anim Pract 2010;51:113–8.
10. Plunkett SJ. Urogenital and reproductive emergencies. In: Emergency procedures for the small animal veterinarian. 2nd edition. London: WB Saunders; 2001. p. 211–48.
11. Linde-Forsberg C, Walett Darvelid A. Dystocia in the bitch: a retrospective study of 182 cases. J Sm Anim Pract 2008;35:402–7.
12. Barber J. Parturition and dystocia. In: Root-Kustritz MV, editor. Small animal theriogenology. London: Butterworth/Heinemann; 2003. p. 241–79.
13. Smith FO. Challenges in small animal parturition: timing elective and emergency cesarian sections. Theriogenology 2007;68:348–53.
14. Pretzer SD. Medical management of canine and feline dystocia. Theriogenology 2008;70:333–6.
15. Davidson AP. Primary uterine inertia in four Labrador bitches. J Am Anim Hosp Assoc 2011;47:83–8.
16. Gunn-Moore DA, Ridyard AE, Welsh EA. Succesful treatment of uterine torsion in a cat with severe metabolic and haemostatic complications. J Feline Med Surg 2000; 2:115–9.
17. Pacchiana PD, Stanley SW. Uterine torsion and metabolic abnormalities in a cat with pyometra. Can Vet J 2008;49:398–400.
18. Reiss AJ. Dystocia. In: Veterinary emergency medicine secrets. 2nd ed. Philadelphia: Hanley & Belfus; 2001. p. 370–4.
19. Blaze CA, Glowaski MM. Cesarean section in dogs and cats. In: Veterinary anesthesia drug quick reference. St Louis: Elsevier Saunders; 2004. p. 226–9.
20. Traas AM. Surgical management of canine and feline dystocia. Theriogenology 2008;70:337–42.
21. Traas AM. Resuscitation of canine and feline neonates. Theriogenology 2008;70: 343–8.

Clinical Approach to Abortion, Stillbirth, and Neonatal Death in Dogs and Cats

Catherine G. Lamm, DVM, MRCVS[a,*], Bradley L. Njaa, DVM, MVSc[b]

KEYWORDS

• Abortion • Diagnostics • Neonatal • Stillbirth

The normal gestational period for the dog is 57 to 72 days and that for the cat is between 52 and 74 days.[1,2] Fetal death during gestation can result in resorption, expulsion (abortion), or fetal retention and mummification.[3] If the neonate is born dead at full term, it is stillborn. Neonatal death is considered to be death within the first 3 weeks after birth. Diagnostic procedures to determine the cause of abortion, stillbirth, or neonatal death in dogs and cats are relatively similar in terms of sample collection and submission. For diagnosis, it is critical to collect the appropriate samples, including representative fetal tissues, fetal and maternal blood samples as well as placenta, for further ancillary testing.

When initially presented with an aborted, stillborn, or dead neonatal puppy or kitten, contact the local veterinary diagnostic laboratory prior to sample collection and submission. As all diagnostic laboratories vary, your local diagnostic laboratory will be able to advise you on their preferred sample types and methods of submission. Regional diagnostic laboratories often have abortion panels with discount rates and occasionally have abortion kits available to assist you in sample collection. This information may be useful as you work through the case.

The purpose of this article is to provide a guide to the investigation of abortion, stillbirth, and neonatal death in dogs and cats. It focuses on diagnostic procedures, differentials, and ancillary testing in these species.

The authors have nothing to disclose.

[a] School of Veterinary Medicine, University of Glasgow, Bearsden, Glasgow, G61 1QH, UK
[b] Department of Pathobiology, Oklahoma State University, Stillwater, OK 74076, USA
* Corresponding author.
E-mail address: Catherine.Lamm@glasgow.ac.uk

Vet Clin Small Anim 42 (2012) 501–513
doi:10.1016/j.cvsm.2012.01.015 vetsmall.theclinics.com

DIAGNOSTIC PROCEDURES FOR ABORTION, STILLBIRTH, AND NEONATAL DEATH IN DOGS AND CATS

One of the greatest challenges of the diagnostic procedure is obtaining appropriate samples. Dogs and cats frequently eat the placenta and will occasionally consume dead fetuses as well. The placenta is the most critical tissue to obtain and can have more diagnostic value than the fetus itself.[4] Submission of fetuses/deceased neonates, placenta, and serum from the dam is ideal. Early submission and proper storage and transport of samples are critical to prevent tissue autolysis, which can inhibit both histopathologic interpretation and ancillary testing.[4] In outbreak situations within kennels or catteries, submission of acute and convalescent serum samples from affected and unaffected bitches or queens is extremely useful in tracking infections as they progress through the population.

The procedure outlined later for evaluation of fetal or neonatal death is a guideline. Please contact your local diagnostic laboratory for their preferred samples and testing methods. **Fig. 1** provides a check-off list to help you through the work-up of abortion or stillbirth cases.

A complete history is integral in determining the cause of abortion or neonatal death. Submissions should be accompanied by a complete history, which includes:

- Is the bitch/queen primiparous or multiparous?
- What is the size of the litter and number of littermates affected?
- Has the bitch of queen had problems with previous litters? If so, what diagnostic testing was completed?
- Are there other animals in the household? Are they used for breeding?
- Have other bitches/queens in the household experienced any other reproductive problems including infertility, abortion, or stillbirths? If so, what were they and were any diagnostic procedures performed?
- Do any other animals in the home have upper respiratory disease, diarrhea, or other clinical signs?
- What is the vaccination history of bitch/queen?
- What is the health status of the dam and surviving littermates?
- What is the breeding history of the bitch/queen and stud/tom?
- Has any genetic testing been completed?
- Have there been new additions to the household or kennel/cattery? Have any dogs/cats in the household travelled and returned recently? What quarantine protocols are implemented?

With this information, the diagnostician can target diagnostic testing and make further suggestions as needed if the standard diagnostic tests results are negative.

When presented with a dead fetus or neonate, the animal may be forwarded as a whole carcass to the diagnostic laboratory. Alternatively, the submitting veterinarian can perform a necropsy with appropriate samples collected and shipped. When submitting samples, record any gross abnormalities observed on the general accession form and, ideally, capture a few gross images as part of the submission. However, rarely will gross lesions be observed even when infectious causes are suspected. Because of this it is critical to collect samples for histopathology, serology, bacteriology, and virology in order to attempt to identify a cause. If a fungal disease is suspected, fungal cultures usually need to be specifically requested on the submission form as not all fungal organisms will grow on routine aerobic cultures. Definitive diagnosis is not always achieved but this testing scheme will help rule out infectious causes.

Check-off List for Feline and Canine Abortion, Stillbirth, and Neonatal Death

1. Completed Submission Form

- ☐ Complete history including any lesions noted

2. In Blood Tube for Serology

- ☐ Dam serum
- ☐ Serum or fetal fluid

3. In Formalin for Histopathology

Thin (less than 0.5 cm wide) sections of the following:

- ☐ Placenta
- ☐ Liver
- ☐ Kidney
- ☐ Lung
- ☐ Heart
- ☐ Brain
- ☐ Any lesions, specify on form

4. Fresh for Virology and Bacteriology

- ☐ Placenta
- ☐ Lung (fetuses only)
- ☐ Liver
- ☐ Kidney
- ☐ Spleen (neonates only)
- ☐ Any lesions, specify on form

5. In Blood Tube for Culture

- ☐ Stomach contents (fetuses only)

Fig. 1. Check-off list to assist in sample collection on cases of fetal or neonatal death.

Necropsy

Assemble necessary tools for a necropsy prior to starting, including a scalpel, scissors, forceps, needles, syringes, blood tubes with no additives, and collection

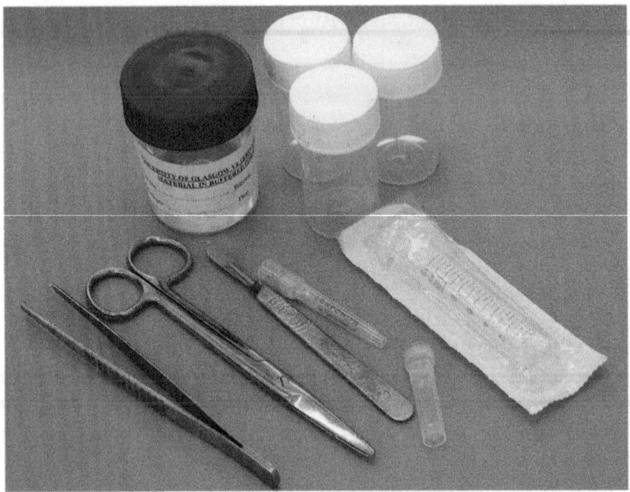

Fig. 2. Minimum supplies needed for a complete postmortem examination of a puppy or kitten.

containers for both histopathology and microbiological testing (**Fig. 2**). Measure and record the animal's weight. If a fetus or other animal that has died within 24 to 48 hours of birth, measure the crown-to-rump length. Document amount of hair growth present and whether it is soft or coarse. Toward the end of gestation, teeth should erupt through the gums. In aggregate, weight, crown-to-rump length, level of hair growth and its texture, and the presence or absence of erupted teeth will help define gestational age.

Rinse any fecal or other material from the fetus and fetal membranes and place on a wet table to begin the examination. Carefully perform a detailed external examination looking for abnormalities, including congenital defects, such as palatoschisis, spina bifida, and limb abnormalities or skull abnormalities. Examine the head and limbs for any evidence of redness, swelling, or improper mobility that may indicate a fracture or other musculoskeletal disease. Examine the umbilicus for evidence of swelling or redness that may indicate inflammation or bulging that may indicate an umbilical hernia.

Use a scalpel to reflect the limbs and open the thoracic and abdominal cavities (**Fig. 3**). With the cavities opened and prior to more thoroughly examining the internal organs, aseptically collect samples for bacteriology and virology testing as outlined in **Fig. 1**. Clean scissors, forceps, and a new scalpel blade should be used for collection. If possible, dip the instruments in alcohol and allow to air dry or flame prior to collection of samples. Do not touch the samples with your gloves or allow the sample to come in contact with anything other than your collection tools and the inside of the collection jar. The samples should be at least 1 cm^3 for bacteriology and virology. Collect heart blood and stomach contents using separate sterile syringes with needles and inject directly into separate blood collection tubes without additives. If heart blood cannot be aspirated, collect any free fluid within the abdominal or thoracic cavity (fetal fluid) and submit that for serology as an alternative. Samples for histopathology will be collected later.

Once all of the cavities have been opened and aseptic samples have been collected, examine the carcass for evidence of any gross lesions. Pay particular

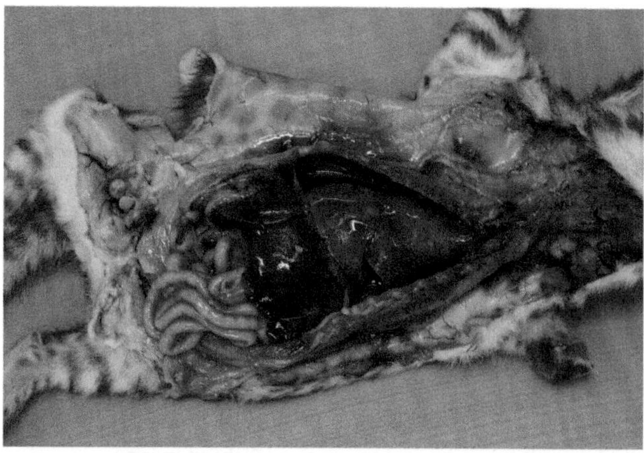

Fig. 3. Abdominal and thoracic cavities of a neonatal kitten opened for postmortem examination. (*Photograph taken by and courtesy of* Richard Irvine.)

attention to hemorrhages, both internal and external, as well as congenital defects such as a ventricular septal defect within the heart. Representative samples should be taken from all organs examined for histopathology and should be less than 0.5 cm in width for proper fixation. Samples should be placed in 10% neutral buffered formalin in a sealable contained with a 1:10 ratio of tissue to formalin to ensure proper fixation. Be aware that the pathologist will often only examine a fraction of the organs collected as they will target specific areas based on species, history, and gross findings.

To examine the placenta, rinse gently with tap water and spread the membranes out on a flat surface. Dogs and cats have a zonary placenta. In dogs, the placenta is often bordered by dark red to dark green bands, which correspond to areas of hemorrhage (**Fig. 4**). This is a normal anatomic structure known as the marginal or

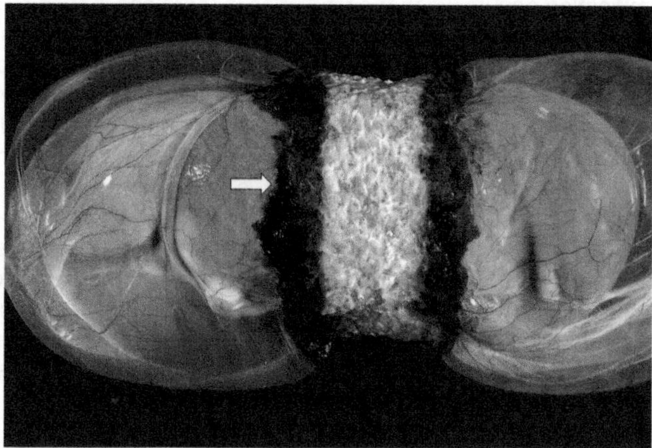

Fig. 4. Chorioallantois of a dog. Note the dark red to green bands representing the marginal hematomas on either side of the zonary placental attachment (*arrow*). The fetus can be seen within the fetal membranes.

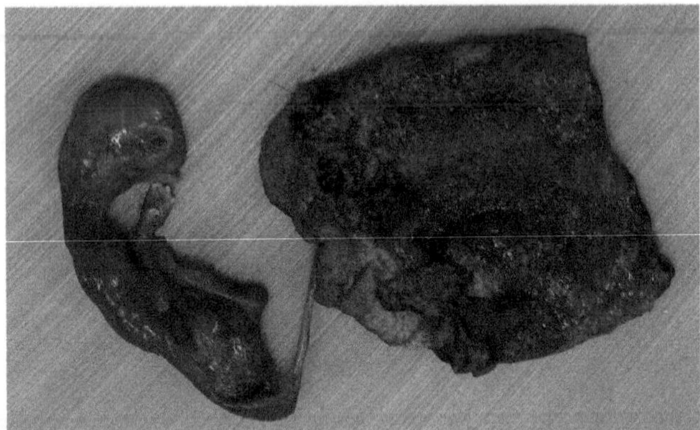

Fig. 5. Mummified aborted fetal kitten and placenta. The fetus has a shrunken, wrinkled appearance. (*Photograph taken by and courtesy of* Richard Irvine.)

perizonal hematoma. This structure is much narrower and less distinct in cats and is pale brown. Any abnormalities in the placenta should be noted and a sample collected for histopathology. An impression smear of the chorioallantois should be obtained in order to examine for evidence of inflammatory cells and/or bacterial organisms. *Brucella* organisms are particularly evident within placental impression smears, allowing for rapid diagnosis. A section of placenta should also be collected for bacterial culture as earlier described.

Assigning Significance to Gross Findings

Some findings within the fetus may appear grossly striking but are incidental. It is common for fetuses to have a red tinge to their internal organs. Only when well-demarcated areas of obvious hemorrhage and/or edema are present is the lesion clinically relevant. Clear yellow or red fluid may be present within the body cavities as an incidental finding. The presence of clotted blood within the cavities is not normal, however, and may indicate trauma.

Fetal mummification occurs when the fetus dies in utero and is then retained for an extended period of time. The fetus will appear dry and shrunken and have wrinkled skin (**Fig. 5**). This is a nonspecific change that can be seen with viral infection as well as many other causes of in utero death. This change is in stark contrast to fetal maceration, which commonly occurs with bacterial infections, as the bacteria continue to replicate within the dead fetus, resulting in gas production and quick degradation of the fetal tissues. The end result is typically fetal bones mixed with reddish brown uterine fluid.

Congenital defects, such as those mentioned earlier, can be seen at necropsy and gross examination is often the only way to diagnose abnormalities such as heart defects. Congenital defects can cause fetal or neonatal death, such as hydranceph-aly, or can be incidental, such as with unilateral renal agenesis. If you are unsure if a lesion is related to the death of the animal, take a photograph, write a detailed description, and send it to a pathologist for consultation.

Preparing Your Submission

Package the formalin container in a separate plastic bag from the fresh tissues and serum. Make sure absorbent material is present in this plastic bag to prevent leakage and contamination. Fill out the appropriate paperwork for your diagnostic laboratory. On the submission form, be sure to include all findings on necropsy examination as well as the information required for a detailed history as mentioned earlier. Submission of digital or scanned images is encouraged.

Again, check whether the local diagnostic laboratory offers an abortion profile. If an abortion profile is not offered, request the following:

- Aerobic, *Campylobacter*, and *Salmonella* cultures of the lung and liver (pooled), stomach contents, and placenta
- Herpesvirus polymerase chain reaction (PCR) on the kidney if renal hemorrhages are noted grossly
- Serology for herpesvirus, brucellosis (dog only), and leptospirosis
- Histopathology of formalin fixed tissues.

Ship the samples overnight on ice packs. Call your regional diagnostic laboratory to see if they are open on Saturday before shipping overnight on a Friday. Fresh samples should be stored at 4°C until submission is possible. If samples must be stored for more than 3 days, freeze the fresh samples and store the formalin-fixed tissues at room temperature until the samples can be shipped. When concerned about anaerobic bacterial infections, make sure to use appropriate swabs and store them in anaerobic storage containers at room temperature until shipment. Never freeze tissues for histopathology as this causes severe artifactual tissue destruction.

If concerned about a genetic disease, there are numerous referral laboratories that offer different genetic tests. One example is the Veterinary Genetics Laboratory at the University of California, Davis, which offers a wide variety of test options in the dog and cat. Most testing is done from blood samples. However, contact the referral laboratory directly to discuss required samples and shipping requirements for the particular test requested.

Maternal causes of abortion and neonatal death are broad and require an extensive work-up by the veterinarian. In addition to routine testing, hormone levels, endometrial biopsies, and other diagnostic procedures in the bitch and queen are available. More information on evaluation of the bitch, is available in detail in article by Wilborn and Maxwell elsewhere in this issue.

Interpretation of Results

Each diagnostic test offered by a laboratory has the potential for both false-positive and false-negative results. As with diagnostic testing in the live animal, each result should be interpreted within the context of the clinical findings and gross or histologic abnormalities. Interpretation of serology results is particularly precarious as a positive result may only indicate exposure or vaccination rather than true infection and cause of abortion or neonatal death. If you have questions about interpretation of results, contact the specialists at the diagnostic laboratory for further explanation.

DIFFERENTIALS FOR ABORTION, STILLBIRTH, AND NEONATAL DEATH IN DOGS AND CATS

The causes of fetal and neonatal loss can be broadly separated into infectious and noninfectious etiologies.[3–5] The main purpose of diagnostic evaluations in the fetus and neonate is to rule out infectious disease and significant congenital defects as causes of abortion. Infectious disease is particularly critical to rule out as this may affect other litters within large-scale breeding operations. Trauma either from delivery or following birth can also result in death in dogs and cats. Other noninfectious

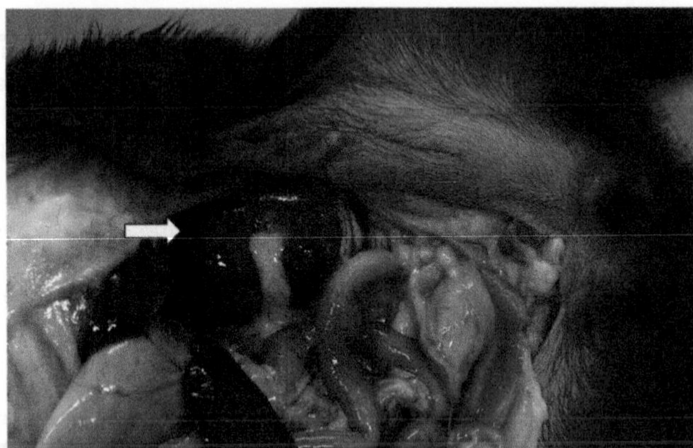

Fig. 6. Neonatal puppy with herpesvirus infection. There are hemorrhages within the kidney (*arrow*). (*Photograph taken by and courtesy of* Richard Irvine.)

causes, including genetic disease and maternal factors, are much more difficult to diagnose.[4,5] Once infectious diseases, trauma, and congenital defects have been ruled out, the possibility of maternal factors as a cause should be explored clinically. For additional information on infertility in the bitch, please see article by Wilborn and Maxwell elsewhere in this issue.

Infectious Causes

Infectious causes of abortion in dogs and cats can be broadly grouped into viral, bacterial, fungal, and protozoal diseases. The diagnostic protocol proposed in this chapter attempts to identify infection with a particular organism, targeting the most common causes of fetal and neonatal death in the United States. This protocol does not include testing for less common etiologies, such as *Leishmania* spp and bluetongue virus (BTV).[6,7]

The most common cause of viral abortion and neonatal death in dogs is herpesviral infection.[8–11] Puppies can be infected in utero or at the time of parturition and death can occur in utero or up to 3 weeks following birth.[12] Body temperature plays an important role in neonatal herpesviral mortality, with viral replication optimized at lower temperatures.[12] Clinical presentations include sudden death, lethargy, and excessive crying.[12] Herpesviral infection in dogs is usually easy to diagnose on postmortem examination and is characterized by multiorgan haemorrhages, the most notable of which are seen in the kidney, lung, and liver (**Fig. 6**).[12] Herpesviral infection can be confirmed with histopathology and polymerase chain reaction. In cats, herpesviral infection as a cause of abortion is extremely rare and is most often associated with respiratory disease in the queen rather than direct infection of the fetus.[13] As in dogs, neonatal death due to herpesvirus can be seen in kittens.[10] For more information on herpesviral infection in dogs, please see article by Decaro and colleagues elsewhere in this issue.

Other viral infections known to cause sporadic abortions and neonatal death in dogs include BTV, canine parvovirus-1 (canine minute virus), canine distemper virus (CDV), and canine adenovirus-1 (CAV1).[10,14] Fetal and/or neonatal death may be secondary to maternal morbidity or due to direct infection.[10] BTV and canine parvovirus-1 infection are covered in detail in article by Decaro and colleagues elsewhere in this issue. Abortions associated with CDV are rare and most often associated with maternal morbidity. In a small percentage of cases, the virus can cross the placenta and result in direct fetal infection.[15] CAV1 is not typically associated with abortion; however, CAV1 infection has been associated with fatal pneumonia in pups less than 4 weeks of age.[16]

Causes of sporadic viral abortion and neonatal death in cats include feline leukemia virus, feline parvovirus (feline panleukopenia virus), feline immunodeficiency virus, feline coronavirus, and feline calicivirus (FCaV).[10,13,16–20] Most of these viral infections are covered in detail in article by Decaro and colleagues elsewhere in this issue. FCaV infection in the queen can result in abortion secondary to maternal morbidity. Rarely, FCaV can cross the placenta, resulting in fetal infection, widespread cutaneous hemorrhages within the fetus, and subsequent abortion.[18]

The two most common causes of bacterial abortion and neonatal death in dogs are *Brucella canis* and *Streptococcus* spp infection.[3,21–24] Additional information on these organisms is provided in article by Graham and Taylor elsewhere in this issue. Infection with other bacterial organisms, such as *Escherichia coli*, *Campylobacter* spp, *Leptospira* spp, and *Salmonella* spp can occur sporadically.[3,25–27] Most bacterial causes of abortion and neonatal death will be isolated during routine aerobic cultures.[26] Although *Brucella* spp will grow on routine blood agar plates, colonies often take several days to become visible. Because of this, routine cultures that are reported as "no growth" at 48 hours have not ruled out brucellosis. Other exceptions include *Salmonella* spp and *Campylobacter* spp, both of which require special culture techniques. *Leptospira* spp are extremely difficult to culture, and growth can take several weeks. Paired serology on blood from the bitch or queen is a rapid diagnostic tool for leptospirosis. It is important to remember that recent vaccination of the dam may interfere with serologic interpretation. Histopathology is recommended to confirm that the organisms isolated from routine bacterial cultures are indeed associated with an infectious process and not a contaminant. This is particularly true concerning isolates from the placentas it is often contaminated by feces and other material that may be present in the birthing area. Bacterial causes of abortion in cats are similar to those in dogs, with the exception of brucellosis.[13,17,28,29] Abortions due to fungal infection are rare in dogs and cats.

Although protozoal infections may result in abortion, stillbirth, or neonatal death in dogs and cats, it is extremely rare. Cats and dogs are the definitive hosts for the protozoa *Toxoplasma gondii* and *Neospora caninum*, respectively.[3,30] Cats and dogs can serve as a source of infection in other animals with these organisms, which can result in abortion in other species, particularly ruminants and people.[30] Cats harboring *T gondii* are typically asymptomatic, although immune-suppressed cats can develop systemic toxoplasmosis particularly when infected with virulent strains, which can result in significant morbidity and mortality.[13,31] If the queen has systemic toxoplasmosis, she may abort due to systemic illness rather than direct fetal infection.[3,13,32] Transplacental transmission and fetal infection with *T gondii* have been shown in cats and dogs experimentally and associated fetal death has been reported.[3,31,33] Abortion or stillbirth related to neosporosis in dogs and cats has not been reported.[3,34]

Traumatic Causes

Traumatic causes of abortion in dogs and cats can be further subdivided into trauma during parturition, such as with dystocia, and trauma occurring after birth.[35] Dystocia is often noted by the owner during parturition. Affected puppies or kittens often have regionally extensive hemorrhage and/or edema. Location of the lesions varies and is

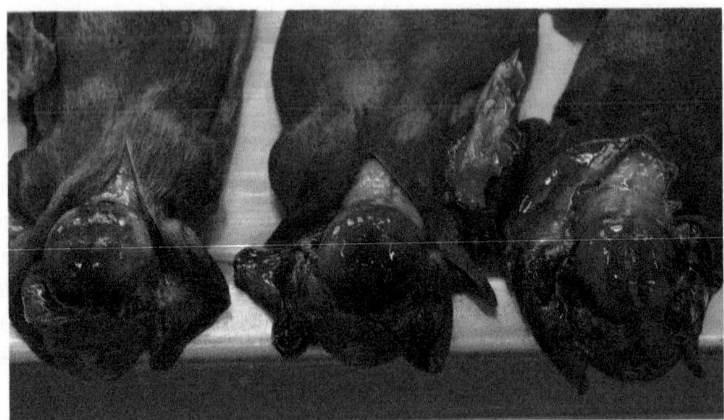

Fig. 7. Three neonatal puppies from the same litter. There is extensive hemorrhage around and within the skull, typical of infanticide. (*Photograph taken by and courtesy of* Richard Irvine.)

dependent upon where the fetus was lodged within the birth canal and for how long. Other puppies or kittens within the litter may or may not be affected. Following cases of dystocia, the mother should be evaluated for possible causes of dystocia and cesarean section delivery may be considered in future pregnancies.

Neonatal trauma is often characterized by regionally extensive hemorrhage that may be accompanied by fractures of bones within the affected area. Infanticide is often caused by skull crushing and results in hemorrhage and fractures of the skull (**Fig. 7**). In cases of infanticide, typically more than one puppy or kitten in the litter may be affected. Dams that commit infanticide in one litter are at increased risk of committing infanticide in future litters.

Congenital Defects and Genetic Disorders

Congenital defects can be sporadic and without direct cause, can be a phenotypic reflection of a genetic disease, or can be related to toxin ingestion.[5,13,35] If similar congenital defects are present in more than one animal in the litter, further workup is required to rule out the 2 latter causes. Chromosomal defects typically result in early embryonic death and resorption.[10,13] As mentioned previously, referral laboratories are your best resources for confirming genetic disorders and should be contacted directly for submission guidelines.

Noninfectious Causes and Maternal Factors

The potential for abortion and stillbirth always exists if the bitch or queen is systemically ill, is excessively stressed, has received severe trauma, is administered certain drugs, ingests certain toxins, etc.[5,10,35,36] Once infectious and traumatic causes of abortion, stillbirth, and neonatal death have been ruled out, the possibility of maternal morbidity as the cause for fetal or neonatal death should be explored.

Abnormalities in metabolism or nutrition, such as diabetes mellitus, hypothyroidism, eclampsia, and pregnancy toxemia, can result in fetal or neonatal loss in the bitch and queen.[13,21,32,37] Diabetes mellitus in the bitch has been associated with fetal loss and stillbirths.[21] Due to persistent hyperglycemia, puppies born to bitches with diabetes are often large and dystocia can occur.[21] Pregnancy toxemia occurs secondary to a negative energy balance related to large litter sizes and/or inadequate food intake.[21] Eclampsia is characterized by low serum calcium, which can result in fetal loss in the bitch and the queen.[13,32] Clinical chemistries and urinalysis are helpful in diagnosing diabetes, pregnancy toxaemia, and eclampsia.[21]

Hypoluteinization occurs when the corpra lutei secrete insufficient progesterone to maintain pregnancy and has been reported in dogs.[3,10,38–41] Typically, these dogs appear clinically infertile due to recurrent early embryonic loss and resorption.[41] Hypoluteinization can be a treatable disease that is diagnosed by measurement of serum progesterone levels.[3,41]

Other Causes of Neonatal Death

Following birth, some kittens and puppies fail to thrive and are often lumped together using the phrase "fading syndrome."[42] As the name implies, fading syndrome is used to simply describe a clinical presentation rather than a specific etiology.[42] This syndrome can be caused by a wide variety of infectious, toxic, traumatic, metabolic, and genetic diseases.[42] Maternal factors, such as mastitis, may also play a role. The cause for the fading syndrome may be readily evident, such as with a cleft palate and inability to effectively nurse, or may be much more obscure, such as idiopathic hypoglycemia resulting in hepatic lipidosis.[26] A complete postmortem examination of the affected neonate and thorough physical examination of the dam and littermates are required to determine the cause of failure to thrive.

SUMMARY

Diagnosis of the cause of abortion, stillbirth, and neonatal death in the dog and cat can be challenging. The purpose of the diagnostic procedures outlined in this article is to provide the practitioner with a protocol for collection of quality samples and a guide to the recommended ancillary testing. The purpose of this procedure is to explore potential infectious causes of abortion and limit the spread of disease within a kennel population. Other sporadic causes of death may be more difficult to diagnose. Ultimately, it is important that the regional diagnostic laboratory be contacted prior to sample collection to ensure optimal results.

REFERENCES

1. Johnston SD, Root Kustritz MV, Olson PN. Feline pregnancy. In: Canine and feline theriogenology. Philadelphia: Saunders; 2001. p. 421.
2. Johnston SD, Root Kustritz MV, Olson PN. Canine pregnancy. In: Canine and feline theriogenology. Philadelphia: Saunders; 2001. p. 76.
3. Pretzer SD. Bacterial and protozoal causes of pregnancy loss in the bitch and queen. Theriogenology 2008;70:320–6.
4. Schlafer DH. Canine and feline abortion diagnostics. Theriogenology 2008;70: 327–31.
5. Johnston SD, Raksil S. Fetal loss in the dog and cat. Vet Clin North Am Small Anim Pract 1987;17:535–54.
6. Wilbur LA, Evermann JF, Levings RL, et al. Abortion and death in pregnant bitches associated with a canine vaccine contaminated with bluetongue virus. J Am Vet Med Assoc 1994;204:1762–5.
7. Dubey JP, Rosypal AC, Pierce V, et al. Placentitis associated with leishmaniasis in a dog. J Am Vet Med Assoc 2005;227:1266–9, 50.
8. Dahlbom M, Johnsson M, Myllys V, et al. Seroprevalence of canine herpesvirus-1 and Brucella canis in finnish breeding kennels with and without reproductive problems. Reprod Domest Anim 2009;44:128–31.

9. Ronsse V, Verstegen J, Onclin K, et al. Risk factors and reproductive disorders associated with canine herpesvirus-1 (CHV-1). Theriogenology 2004;61:619–36.
10. Verstegen J, Dhaliwal G, Verstegen-Onclin K. Canine and feline pregnancy loss due to viral and non-infectious causes: a review. Theriogenology 2008;70:304–19.
11. Ronsse V, Verstegen J, Thiry E, et al. Canine herpesvirus-1 (CHV-1): clinical, serological and virological patterns in breeding colonies. Theriogenology 2005;64:61–74.
12. Hashimoto A, Hirai K, Yamaguchi T, et al. Experimental transplacental infection of pregnant dogs with canine herpesvirus. Am J Vet Res 1982;43:844–50.
13. Root Kustritz MV. Clinical management of pregnancy in cats. Theriogenology 2006; 66:145–50.
14. Carmichael LE, Schlafer DH, Hashimoto A. Pathogenicity of minute virus of canines (MVC) for the canine fetus. Cornell Vet 1991;81:151–71.
15. Krakowka S, Hoover EA, Koestner A, et al. Experimental and naturally occurring transplacental transmission of canine distemper virus. Am J Vet Res 1977;38: 919–22.
16. Almes KM, Janardhan KS, Anderson J, et al. Fatal canine adenoviral pneumonia in two litters of bulldogs. J Vet Diagn Invest 2010;22:780–4.
17. Romagnoli S. Clinical approach to infertility in the queen. J Feline Med Surg 2003;5: 143–6.
18. van Vuuren M, Geissler K, Gerber D, et al. Characterisation of a potentially abortigenic strain of feline calicivirus isolated from a domestic cat. Vet Rec 1999;144:636–8.
19. Weaver CC, Burgess SC, Nelson PD, et al. Placental immunopathology and pregnancy failure in the FIV-infected cat. Placenta 2005;26:138–47.
20. Cave TA, Thompson H, Reid SW, et al. Kitten mortality in the United Kingdom: a retrospective analysis of 274 histopathological examinations (1986 to 2000). Vet Rec 2002;151:497–501.
21. Root Kustritz MV. Pregnancy diagnosis and abnormalities of pregnancy in the dog. Theriogenology 2005;64:755–65.
22. Gyuranecz M, Szeredi L, Ronai Z, et al. Detection of Brucella canis-induced reproductive diseases in a kennel. J Vet Diagn Invest 2011;23:143–7.
23. Hollett RB. Canine brucellosis: outbreaks and compliance. Theriogenology 2006;66: 575–87.
24. Lamm CG, Ferguson AC, Lehenbauer TW, et al. Streptococcal infection in dogs: a retrospective study of 393 cases. Vet Pathol 2010;47:387–95.
25. Redwood DW, Bell DA. Salmonella panama: isolation from aborted and newborn canine fetuses. Vet Rec 1983;112:362.
26. Munnich A. The pathological newborn in small animals: the neonate is not a small adult. Vet Res Commun 2008;32(Suppl 1):81–5.
27. Linde C. Partial abortion associated with genital Escherichia coli infection in a bitch. Vet Rec 1983;112:454–5.
28. Reilly GA, Bailie NC, Morrow WT, et al. Feline stillbirths associated with mixed Salmonella typhimurium and Leptospira infection. Vet Rec 1994;135:608.
29. Hoskins JD. Feline neonatal sepsis. Vet Clin North Am Small Anim Pract 1993;23:91–100.
30. Bandini LA, Neto AF, Pena HF, et al. Experimental infection of dogs (Canis familiaris) with sporulated oocysts of Neospora caninum. Vet Parasitol 2011;176:151–6.
31. Sakamoto CA, da Costa AJ, Gennari SM, et al. Experimental infection of pregnant queens with two major Brazilian clonal lineages of Toxoplasma gondii. Parasitol Res 2009;105:1311–6.
32. Wiebe VJ, Howard JP. Pharmacologic advances in canine and feline reproduction. Top Comp Anim Med 2009;24:71–99.

33. Bresciani KD, Costa AJ, Toniollo GH, et al. Transplacental transmission of Toxoplasma gondii in reinfected pregnant female canines. Parasitol Res 2009;104:1213–7.
34. Barber JS, Trees AJ. Naturally occurring vertical transmission of Neospora caninum in dogs. Int J Parasitol 1998;28:57–64.
35. Bucheler J. Fading kitten syndrome and neonatal isoerythrolysis. Vet Clin North Am Small Anim Pract 1999;29:853–70, v.
36. Dieter JA, Stewart DR, Haggarty MA, et al. Pregnancy failure in cats associated with long-term dietary taurine insufficiency. J Reprod Fertil Suppl 1993;47:457–63.
37. Panciera DL, Purswell BJ, Kolster KA. Effect of short-term hypothyroidism on reproduction in the bitch. Theriogenology 2007;68:316–21.
38. Gorlinger S, Galac S, Kooistra HS, et al. Hypoluteoidism in a bitch. Theriogenology 2005;64:213–9.
39. Johnson CA. Disorders of pregnancy. Vet Clin North Am Small Anim Pract 1986;16:477–82.
40. Tibold A, Thuroczy J. Progesterone, oestradiol, FSH and LH concentrations in serum of progesterone-treated pregnant bitches with suspected luteal insufficiency. Reprod Domest Anim 2009;44(Suppl 2):129–32.
41. Johnson CA. High-risk pregnancy and hypoluteoidism in the bitch. Theriogenology 2008;70:1424–30.
42. Roth JA. Possible association of thymus dysfunction with fading syndromes in puppies and kittens. Vet Clin North Am Small Anim Pract 1987;17:603–16.

Disorders of Sexual Development in Dogs and Cats

Bruce W. Christensen, DVM, MS

KEYWORDS

- Sex determination • Sexual development
- Sex differentiation • Intersex • Gender • DSD

Embryonic and fetal sexual development is often described as sexual determination and differentiation. The *sexual determination* of an individual animal's gender occurs as the sexual genotype of an individual directs the appropriate differentiation of the gonadal tissue, which further influences the *sexual differentiation* of the appropriate accompanying genitalia. This review will give an overview of what is currently known about the normal processes involved in mammalian sexual determination and differentiation and then discuss disorders of sexual development (DSDs) that occur via deviations from the normal pathway. Disorders that have been documented in the dog and cat will be highlighted. What was once considered a relatively simple pathway where the mere presence of a Y chromosome directed male development and the lack of the Y chromosome resulted in the passive development of the female[1] is currently recognized as increasingly more complex.[2–10] Active, ongoing research into sexual development answers more questions and fills in more gaps on a regular basis.

Note that standard genetic nomenclature (http://www.genenames.org)[11] is used throughout this article, as follows: Human gene symbols are in italics and capitalized (*SOX9*). Gene symbols for other vertebrates, such as the dog, are in italics and only the first letter is capitalized (*Sox9*). Protein symbols for vertebrates and humans are in plain text and capitalized (SOX9). Throughout this review, the canine will be used as a model when referring to chromosome counts, unless specifically referring to a feline example.

CHROMOSOMAL SEX

The normal chromosome count for dogs is 78 chromosomes and for cats, 38 chromosomes, including the sex chromosomes. Normal mammalian females have 2 copies of the X chromosome (78,XX in the bitch; 38,XX in the queen), 1 inherited from

The author has nothing to disclose.
Department of Veterinary Clinical Sciences, Iowa State University, 1600 South 16th Street, Ames, IA 50011, USA
E-mail address: drbruce@iastate.edu

Vet Clin Small Anim 42 (2012) 515–526
doi:10.1016/j.cvsm.2012.01.008 **vetsmall.theclinics.com**
0195-5616/12/$ – see front matter

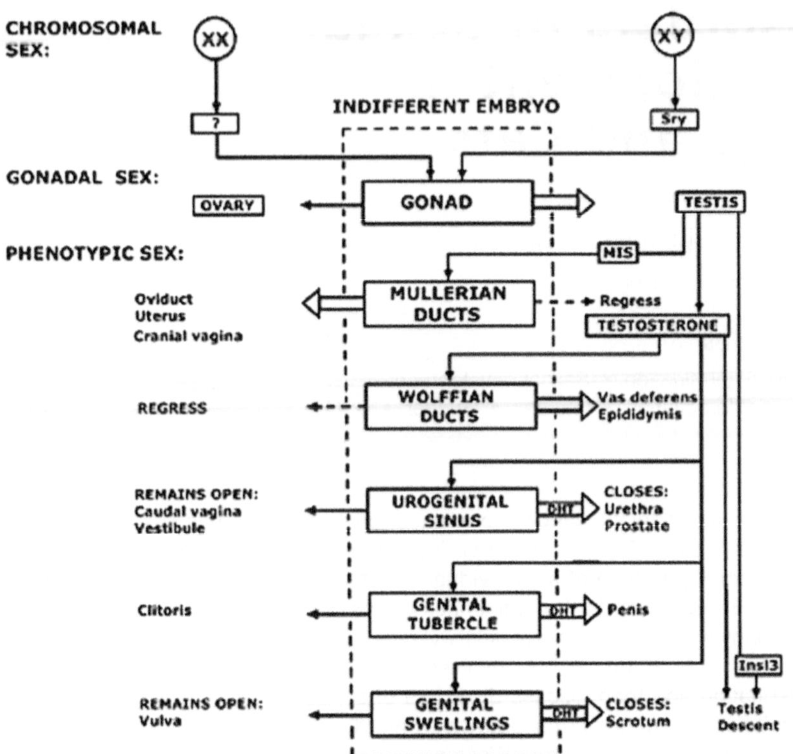

Fig. 1. Overview of normal mammalian sexual development from fertilization to sexual differentiation. (*From* Meyers-Wallen VN. CVT update: inherited disorders of the reproductive tract in dogs and cats. In: Bonagura J, editor. Current veterinary therapy XIV. Philadelphia: WB Saunders; 2008. p. 1034–9; used with permission.)

the dam and 1 from the sire. Normal mammalian males have an X chromosome inherited from the dam and a Y chromosome inherited from the sire (78,XY in the dog; 38,XY in the tom). During the process of meiosis, gametes are produced (oocytes in the female, sperm in the male) that contain only 1 copy of each chromosome of an individual (haploid). Oocytes will contain only 1 of the 2 copies of the X chromosome of the dam. Sperm will contain either the X or Y chromosome from the sire. It is the sperm, therefore, that determines the sex of the individual resulting at conception. If the sperm contains an X chromosome, the ensuing zygote will have a sexual chromosome component of XX and should proceed to develop as a female, whereas if the sperm contains a Y chromosome, the resulting zygote will have a sexual chromosome component of XY and should proceed to develop as a male (**Fig. 1**).

GONADAL SEX

During early embryonic development, both XX and XY individuals initially progress along a common pathway. Early in development, primordial germ cells originating from the lining of the yolk sack migrate to the hindgut and the genital ridge where they reside in the undifferentiated gonad. Primitive sex cords and paired mesonephric (Wolffian) and paramesonephric (Müllerian) ducts form. A summary of known, key

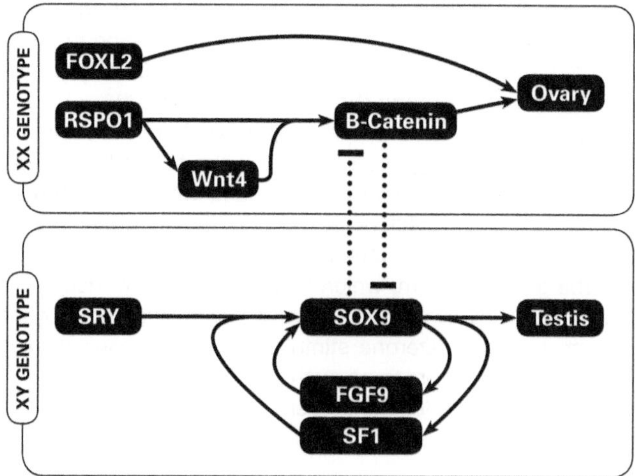

Fig. 2. Overview of genes and their respective proteins involved in sexual determination along the 2 potential paths of the bipotential gonad in mammals. Solid arrows indicate a stimulatory effect; dashed lines with a flat bar indicate an inhibitory relationship.

events of sexual determination and differentiation will be presented here, but as this is an active area of investigation, the reader is encouraged to review recent literature for in-depth and current knowledge on the different roles known genes play in sexual differentiation.[2,3,5–9,12–14]

MALE DIFFERENTIATION

Testicular differentiation in the dog has been observed as early as 36 days of gestation.[15] In the presence of a Y chromosome, the sex-determining region Y chromosome gene (*Sry*) is the initial gene that encodes for the testis-determining factor, which, along with transcription of other genes such as *Sf-1*, initiates an intricate, interactive cascade of genetic signals. SRY seems to act on a single gene, *Sox9*, which activation is continually reinforced by positive feed-forward loops, including an important established relationship with *Fgf9*.[9] In addition to activation by SRY, SF-1 seems to also be necessary to initiate expression of *Sox9*.[14] Both proteins (SRY and SF-1) bind in the same initiator sequence region of *Sox9*.[9] SOX9 then initiates Sertoli cell formation and organization of the sex cords in the embryonic gonad.[16] SRY is only active for a very short window of time (days or hours) during embryogenesis, but SOX9 remains active throughout life inside of the Sertoli cells. SOX9 seems to be able to take the place of SRY in activating *Sox9* alongside SF-1 and FGF9.14 (**Fig. 2**).

While Sertoli cells are differentiating, the sex cords fuse to form a network of medullary sex cords and the rete testes. SOX9 further inhibits the actions of *Wnt4* and *Foxl2*, important genes in the ovarian pathway.[12] The Sertoli cells, under the stimulation of SF-1,[2] secrete Müllerian inhibiting substance (MIS; also known as anti-Müllerian hormone), which induces the regression of the Müllerian ducts.[15] The formation of early Sertoli cells stimulates the differentiation of other cells into Sertoli cells, essentially a positive feedback loop for an initial time. Interstitial cells (Leydig cells) form next and, also due to stimulation from SF-1,[2] secrete testosterone. Testosterone stimulates the Wolffian ducts to mature into the epididymides and vas deferens. The enzyme 5α-reductase converts testosterone into dihydrotestosterone (DHT), which is the primary androgen responsible for stimulating the urogenital sinus to differentiate into the prostate and urethra, the genital tubercle into the penis, and the genital swellings to close to form the scrotum (see **Fig. 1**).

Testicular descent occurs in 3 stages: abdominal translocation, transinguinal migration, and inguinoscrotal migration.[17] Initially, the testes lie in a retroperitoneal position attached to the ligamentous gubernaculum, which runs through the abdomen and the inguinal canal attaching distally to the scrotum. As the abdomen elongates, the cranial suspensory ligament thins and elongates while the testes are held in place by the gubernaculum, which is strengthened by insulin-like peptide 3. Abdominal translocation involves the expression of a number of genes and only partially dependent upon testosterone stimulation.[17] Transinguinal migration is accomplished by intra-abdominal pressure pushing the testes through the inguinal canal (testosterone independent). Under the influence of testosterone, the gubernaculum later regresses, pulling the testes into the final scrotal position.[17]

FEMALE DIFFERENTIATION

Because of lack of knowledge, for many years female differentiation was accepted to be a passive process. While the entire pathway is still not understood, it is now known to be a very active pathway. In the absence of a Y chromosome, and therefore the absence of *Sry*, the balance for gene expression supporting male differentiation (mitigated by *Sox9* and *Fgf9*) and female differentiation (mitigated by *Rspo1* and *Wnt4*) tips in favor of female. *Rspo1*, a gene activated during ovarian development, mediates the activation of *Wnt4* via the β-catenin pathway.[3] SOX9 and β-catenin inactivate each other in the cytoplasm. By a critical point in embryonic development, whichever protein is in excess of the other diffuses into the nucleus and regulates transcription of different genes. Up-regulation of β-catenin supports the transcription of genes necessary for female differentiation, including *Wnt4* (in contrast, deficiency of β-catenin allows SOX9 to support transcription of genes important in male differentiation; see **Fig. 2**).[3]

Suppressor proteins activated in the female pathway prevent activity in the male pathway. WNT4 up-regulates *Dax1*, a gene on the X chromosome that acts in a dose-dependent mode. DAX1 appears to suppress the functions of SF1 in activating *Sox9*, which prevents the stimulation of Sertoli cells to secrete MIS and Leydig cells to secrete testosterone.[2,14] FOXL2 binds to and prevents the activation of *Sox9*.[14] Finally, *Rspo1* also suppresses male differentiation; knocking out *Rspo1* results in seminiferous tubule formation within ovarian tissue.[3]

During ovarian development, cells separate from the sex cords to become granulosa cells. In the absence of Sertoli cells and consequent absence of MIS, no regression signal is sent to the Müllerian ducts. Any specific supportive signals sent from the female pathway have yet to be discovered, but it is known that WNT4 and FOXL2 both support further ovarian differentiation and WNT4 maintains oocyte viability.[2] An abnormal duplication of *Wnt4* in humans caused a male-to-female sex reversal,[18] whereas loss of function of *Wnt4* causes female-to-male sex reversal.[19]

In the absence of Leydig cells and accompanying androgens, the Wolffian ducts regress. The Müllerian ducts develop into the oviducts, uterus, and cranial vagina. In the absence of DHT, the urogenital sinus develops into the caudal vagina and vestibule and the genital tubercle into the clitoris, and the genital swellings remain open and form the vulva (see **Fig. 1**).

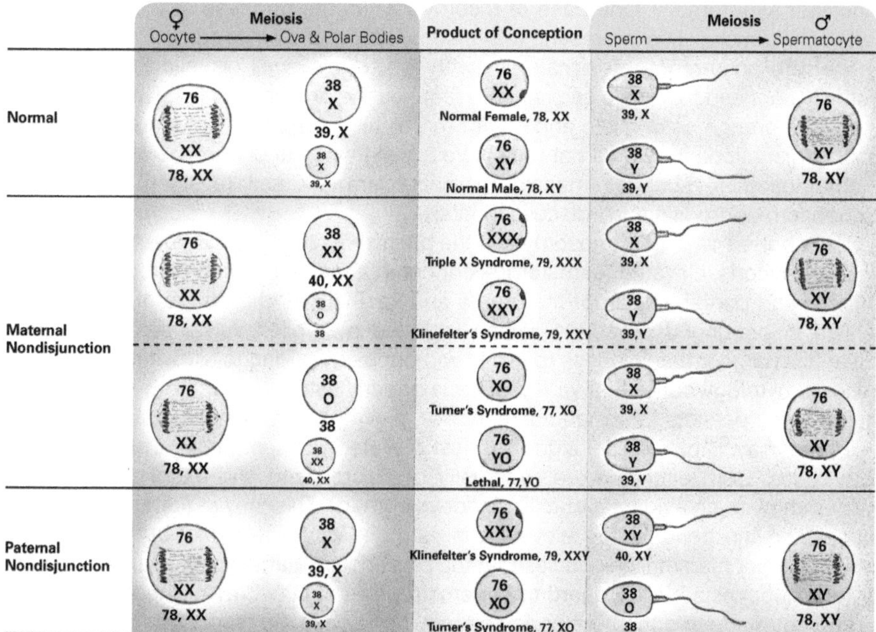

Fig. 3. Overview of normal meiosis and fertilization with respect to sex hormone segregation (*top*) and disorders with consequences that may occur due to nondisjunction events (*lower pathways*) in mammals. *Numbers within cells* indicate the number of *autosomal* chromosomes present alongside the sex chromosomes, which are indicated by an "X" or "Y." *Numbers below cells* indicate the *total number* of chromosomes in the karyotype, autosomal and sex chromosomes inclusive. (*Netter illustration from* netterimages.com.)

DISORDERS OF SEXUAL DEVELOPMENT

Chromosomal Abnormalities

As described, the pathway toward normal development of both the male and female is intricate and deviations at any point tend to result in some type of DSD. In the very early stages, nondisjunction errors during meiosis can result in sex chromosomal abnormalities (**Fig. 3**). Sperm or oocytes that contain an abnormal complement of the sex chromosomes will form either lethal combinations or ones that result in a DSD.

If an oocyte or a spermatozoon lacks a sex chromosome and then fuses with the opposite gamete, which contains an X chromosome, the resultant zygote will have a chromosome count of 77,XO (monosomy X or Turner syndrome).[20] If a sperm or oocyte contains 2 copies of the X chromosome (40,XX), the resultant karyotype after fusion with the opposite gamete, depending on its sex chromosome complement (39,X or 39,Y), will be either 79,XXX or 79,XXY (trisomy X or Klinefelter syndrome, respectively).[21,22] Individuals with sex chromosomal abnormalities tend to have underdeveloped genitalia and be infertile, but the external phenotype tends to be either male (in the case of 79,XXY) or female (in the cases of 77,XO or 79,XXX).

Trisomy XXY (Klinefelter syndrome) has been reported in the dog (79,XXY)[23–25] and the cat (39,XXY).[26] Cases of trisomy XXY have a normal male external phenotype, are associated with infertility due to azoospermia, and have testicular hypoplasia. In humans, cryptorchidism (14%) and gynecomastia (44%) are reported clinical signs of

Klinefelter syndrome.[27] One case of trisomy XXY in the dog was associated with a Sertoli cell tumor.[26] It is interesting that trisomy XXY in the cat is sometimes detected by the rare occurrence of a male cat with the tortoiseshell or calico hair pattern, normally confined to female cats since it requires the presence of 2 X chromosomes, 1 with the orange color allele and 1 with the black color allele. Of course, there are other explanations for why a cat may have a male external phenotype and have two X chromosomes, such as mosaicism, chimerism, XX sex reversal, and female pseudohermaphroditism (all discussed later).

One reported case of monosomy X in the bitch showed signs of hyperandrogenism (enlarged clitoris, elevated testosterone concentrations, decreased estrogen concentrations, and partial aplasia of the uterus and vagina)[28] and 2 others of hyperestrogenism in prolonged proestrus, which included a swollen vulva, serosanguinous vulvar discharge, attractiveness to males without being willing to allow mounting, and a vaginal cytology consistent with proestrus or early estrus.[29,30] In both cases, these clinical signs persisted for months. In 1 case, elevated estrogen was confirmed with a serum assay,[29] but clinical signs suggest elevated concentrations of estrogens in both cases. Both bitches were eventually ovariectomized and examination of the ovaries showed no evidence of follicular development. This may at first be surprising, considering the documented elevation in estrogen concentrations, but it has been shown in other mammalian species that the presence of viable oocytes are necessary for folliculogenesis.[6] With regard to hyperestrogenism, in neither of these cases was an attempt made to document pancytopenia, but 1 case did report a thin hair coat.[29] Both cases reported cystic endometrial hyperplasia, and 1 case reported early signs of pyometra, despite no evidence of elevated progesterone concentrations (and documented baseline concentrations in 1 case[29]).

All reported cases of trisomy X in the bitch have appeared with a normal female external phenotype and have presented for infertility, sometimes with irregular estrous cycles.[31–34] Ovarian functionality in trisomy X bitches varied from persistent anestrus[32] to follicular development without evidence of luteal function[33] to having apparently functional corpora lutea.[34]

Chimerism, which is the consequence of the fusion of 2 zygotes, and mosaicism, which is the consequence of an error in chromosome separation within a certain cell line within 1 embryo, both result in an individual animal that has different chromosome counts in different cell lines.[35] If these errors include the sex chromosomes or chromosomes containing genes important to sexual differentiation, and the cell lines affect the precursors of genital tissues, then a DSD will be the result. Mosaicism resulting in a DSD has been reported in dogs.[30,36–38]

Gonadal Abnormalities

Some dogs with a normal karyotype will develop inappropriate gonadal tissue (78,XX with testicular tissue or 78,XY with ovarian tissue). These individuals have been termed "sex reversals" or more recently have simply been included under the broader category of DSD, as a result of confusion with the definition of "sex reversal" and its consequent improper use,[39] usually in describing pseudohermaphrodites (as in describing dogs with a chromosome count of 78,XY and testicular tissue, but a female external phenotype; see discussion on phenotypic abnormalities later).

One case of an XY true hermaphrodite has been reported in a cat.[40] A 1-year-old cat with the external appearance of a bilaterally cryptorchid tom was presented for neutering. During surgery, it was discovered that the animal had gonads in the region of where the ovaries would be and what appeared to be a bicornuate uterus. Histologic analysis revealed ovotestes and derivatives of both Müllerian and Wolffian duct systems. Karyotyping revealed a normal male chromosome constitution (38,XY), and polymerase chain reaction (PCR) identified the presence of *Sry*. To date, there are no documented cases of true XY sex reversals in dogs. Such a case in a dog would have to demonstrate a chromosome count of 78,XY with the formation of ovarian tissue.

Cases of canine XX sex reversal, a dog with a chromosome count of 78,XX and the formation of testes or ovotestes, have been reported in multiple breeds of dogs,[41,42] but has not yet been reported in cats. XX sex reversal was originally described in the American cocker spaniel.[42] In other breeds an undetermined mode of familial inheritance has been established, but in the American cocker spaniel it has been shown to be inherited in an autosomal recessive fashion.[42] Affected dogs may be XX true hermaphrodites (having ovotestes) or XX males (having only testicular tissue). The degree of masculinization depends on the degree of testicular function, and therefore XX true hermaphrodites may range from having normal female genitalia with limited fertility (some have successfully had litters of puppies) to having an enlarged clitoris and a hypoplastic, infertile female tract. XX males typically are bilaterally cryptorchid and have a caudally displaced prepuce and hypospadias.

A presumptive diagnosis may be made by submitting a tissue sample (usually blood) for karyotyping and using an indirect diagnostic tool such as ultrasonography, palpation, or serum testosterone stimulation assays (human chorionic gonadotropin [hCG] or gonadotropin releasing hormone [GnRH]) to indicate the presence of testicular tissue. Definitive diagnosis requires histopathologic analysis of the gonadal tissue. As part of diagnosis, PCR tests for *Sry* often are performed. In humans, *Sry*-positive XX sex reversal is reported. It is easy to understand that if *Sry* is translocated to the X chromosome, testicular tissue will consequently develop. In the dog, *Sry*-positive XX sex reversal has yet to be reported. More recently, PCR tests and fluorescence in situ hybridization assays for other specific genetic markers in the sexual differentiation pathway are being offered.

Treatment of sex-reversed dogs involves removal of the gonadal or genital tissue if clinical signs accompany the presentation. An enlarged clitoris, for example, may be uncomfortable and predispose the dog to vaginitis. Dogs that have active ovaries may eventually develop a pyometra. Clients should be advised that breeding XX sex-reversed true hermaphrodites is not advised, nor is repeating the breeding of the parents. The trait is almost certainly inherited in all cases, though the exact mode of inheritance has yet to be determined in other breeds. Because the mode of inheritance is not known, a screening test is not yet available and so carrier animals cannot be reliably identified.

Phenotypic Abnormalities

Phenotypic abnormalities considered pseudohermaphrodites occur when the chromosomal and gonadal sex are in agreement but the phenotype disagrees, or is ambiguous. Examples would include a dog with a chromosome constitution of 78,XX, ovaries, and a masculinized external phenotype (female pseudohermaphrodite) or, more commonly, a chromosome constitution of 78,XY, testes (often cryptorchid), and a female external phenotype (male pseudohermaphrodite). These cases are often misdiagnosed as sex reversals and histology of the gonads is usually necessary to tell the difference. Female pseudohermaphrodites can result from the masculinization of female fetuses during development by exposure to endogenous or exogenous progestens or androgens.[43,44]

What may have been male pseudohermaphrodites have been described in the dog,[36,45] although histology of gonadal tissue was not performed and therefore the presence of ovarian tissue (and therefore a diagnosis of sex reversal) could not be ruled out. Two different types of male pseudohermaphroditism have been described and have distinct etiologies: (1) persistent Müllerian duct syndrome (PMDS) and (2) failure of androgen-dependent masculinization.

PMDS is reported in dogs and has been shown to be in higher prevalence in the miniature schnauzer breed, where it is inherited as an autosomal recessive trait.[46–49] Other breeds are less represented, but have been reported.[50,51] Affected dogs are XY males with bilateral testes (approximately half are cryptorchid, either unilateral or bilateral) and androgen-dependent masculinization of both the internal and external genitalia. Alongside the normal internal male genitalia, these males have persistent Müllerian duct derivatives in the form of bilateral oviducts, uterus, cervix, and cranial vagina. Cryptorchid animals may be diagnosed at the time of surgical removal of the cryptorchid testes. Affected animals with scrotal testes are usually not diagnosed until clinical signs of pyometra, urinary tract infection, or prostate disease lead to imaging or surgical diagnostics that identify the Müllerian duct derivatives.[52] Treatment involves surgical removal of the gonads and Müllerian duct derivatives. Prevention involves removing affected and carrier animals from the breeding population. Affected males with descended testes are usually fertile. Carrier animals may be male or female. A molecular test has been developed to diagnose both affected and carrier dogs and it has been proposed to use this test to help eliminate the defect from the breed.[53]

Failure of androgen-dependent masculinization can occur at 3 levels: (1) androgen biosynthesis failure, (2) conversion of testosterone to DHT, and (3) androgen receptor defects. The former 2 etiologies have not been documented in cats or dogs. A defect in the androgen receptor, known to be an X-linked trait, has been documented in both the dog[54] and the cat[55] and is also known as testicular feminization. Affected animals are XY males with bilateral testes but with partial to complete failure of masculinization of the internal and external genitalia. The degree of failure of masculinization is dependent on the degree of loss of function in the androgen receptors. In the case of complete loss of function, the animals will have the external phenotype of a seemingly normal female and present for failure to cycle or otherwise as infertile. Examination will reveal a short, blind-ending vagina with no cervix. There will be no accompanying uterus and gonadal tissue will be purely testicular. Animals with only a partial loss of receptor function will show varying degrees of masculinization. Karyotype will reveal the XY chromosome compliment of a normal male. Androgen assays and androgen stimulation tests will show normal testosterone and DHT production. In the future, androgen receptor assays may be developed to aid in diagnosis. Treatment is castration to avoid the increased incidence of testicular neoplasia in cryptorchid animals. Prevention involves client counseling regarding breeding decisions, keeping in mind that the defect is known to follow X-linked inheritance. Carrier females will be fertile. Litters from carrier females will contain a mixture of genotypes. Half of the females will be carriers, and half of the females will be normal. Half of the males will be affected, and half of the males will be normal. If a litter is already in existence that includes affected males, the most responsible decision would be to not breed any females from that litter, since determining their normal or carrier status is not possible until a genetic test is developed, but breeding normal males from the litter would be acceptable.

Cryptorchidism has understandably been grouped together with other DSDs and isolated cryptorchidism (meaning it is not accompanied by other clinical signs of DSD) is another example of a phenotypic abnormality. The descent of the testes (discussed earlier) is a complicated and incompletely understood process. Testes should be fully descended by 5 days of age in the dog and cat.[56] Descent of the testes after 5 days may occur but should be considered a mild form of cryptorchidism. One study showed that close to 25% of testes in dogs not descended by 10 days would descend later, the majority of which descended by 14 weeks, and none after 6 months of age.[57] Abnormalities at any stage of the process could result in cryptorchidism and therefore noting the location of the cryptorchid testes is useful in understanding the pathogenesis of the condition in a particular patient.

Medical treatments for inducing descent of testes not in the scrotal position by 10 days are anecdotally used by some clinicians, but none have been proved scientifically to work any better in comparison to the 25% that will descend naturally. Potential etiologies of cryptorchidism have been recently reviewed.[17] Complications for cryptorchid testes include an increased incidence of Sertoli cell tumors and seminomas and an increased likelihood for spermatic cord torsion.[58,59] Treatment is bilateral orchidectomy (reviewed recently[60]). While definitive genes for inheritance of cryptorchidism have not been identified, enough data exist to support the conclusion that isolated cryptorchidism is a sex-limited, recessive trait and has a familial inheritance at least in some breeds.[61] As such, both the mother and father of the affected individual should be considered carriers of the trait, as well as some of the full siblings. Prevention involves counseling with clients regarding their breeding program and removing affected dogs and potentially parents and littermates from the breeding program.

SUMMARY

Sex determination and differentiation, whether along the male or female pathway, involves complicated, intricate interactions between different genes, proteins, hormones, and receptors. DSDs occur with deviations at any stage along these pathways. Animals generally present for infertility or evaluation of ambiguous genitalia, but sometimes for other complications such as pyometra or gonadal disease. Definitive diagnosis of the particular type of DSD minimally requires a karyotype, gonadal histology, and description of genital anatomy. Further diagnostic tests to clarify the specific deviation may require PCR, fluorescence in situ hybridization, hormone assays, or receptor assays. Treatment often involves surgical removal of all or part of the reproductive tract but not always. Prevention involves counseling clients with regard to breeding animals, or their relatives, with known heritable disorders.

REFERENCES

1. Jost A, Vigier B, Prepin J, et al. Studies on sex differentiation in mammals. Recent Prog Horm Res 1973;29:1–41.
2. Biason-Lauber A. Control of sex development. Best Pract Res Clin Endocrinol Metab 2010;24:163–86.
3. Chassot AA, Gregoire EP, Magliano M, et al. Genetics of ovarian differentiation: Rspo1, a major player. Sex Dev 2008;2:219–27.
4. DeFalco T, Capel B. Gonad morphogenesis in vertebrates: divergent means to a convergent end. Annu Rev Cell Dev Biol 2009;25:457–82.
5. DiNapoli L, Capel B. SRY and the standoff in sex determination. Mol Endocrinol 2008;22:1–9.
6. Edson MA, Nagaraja AK, Matzuk MM. The mammalian ovary from genesis to revelation. Endocr Rev 2009;30:624–712.
7. Koopman P. The delicate balance between male and female sex determining pathways: potential for disruption of early steps in sexual development. Int J Androl 2010;33:252–8.

8. Piprek RP. Molecular mechanisms underlying female sex determination—antagonism between female and male pathway. Folia Biol 2009;57:105–13.
9. Sekido R, Lovell-Badge R. Sex determination and SRY: down to a wink and a nudge? Trends Genet 2009;25:19–29.
10. Veitia RA. FOXL2 versus SOX9: a lifelong "battle of the sexes." BioEssays 2010;32: 375–80.
11. Wain H, Bruford E, Lovering R, et al. Guidelines for human gene nomenclature. Genomics 2002;79:464–70.
12. Barrionuevo F, Bagheri-Fam S, Klattig J, et al. Homozygous Inactivation of Sox9 causes complete XY sex reversal in mice. Biol Reprod 2006;74:195–201.
13. Blecher SR, Erickson RP. Genetics of sexual development: a new paradigm. Am J Med Genet A 2007;143A:3054–68.
14. Jakob S, Lovell-Badge R. Sex determination and the control of Sox9 expression in mammals. FEBS J 2011;278:1002–9.
15. Meyers-Wallen VN, Manganaro TF, Kuroda T, et al. The critical period for mullerian duct regression in the dog embryo. Biol Reprod 1991;45:626–33.
16. Tilmann C, Capel B. Mesonephric cell migration induces testis cord formation and Sertoli cell differentiation in the mammalian gonad. Development 1999;126:2883–90.
17. Amann RP, Veeramachaneni DNR. Cryptorchidism in common eutherian mammals. Reproduction 2007;133:541–61.
18. Jordan BK, Mohammed M, Ching ST, et al. Up-regulation of WNT-4 signaling and dosage-sensitive sex reversal in humans. Am J Hum Genet 2001;68:1102–9.
19. Mandel H, Shemer R, Borochowitz Z, et al. SERKAL syndrome: an autosomal-recessive disorder caused by a loss-of-function mutation in WNT4. Am J Hum Genet 2008;82:39–47.
20. Kesler SR. Turner syndrome. Child Adolesc Psychiatric Clin North Am 2007;16: 709–22.
21. Tartaglia NR, Howell S, Sutherland A, et al. A review of trisomy X (47,XXX). Orphanet J Rare Dis 2010;5:8.
22. Wikstrom AM, Dunkel L. Klinefelter syndrome. Best Pract Res Clin Endocrinol Metab 2011;25:239–50.
23. Clough E, Pyle RL, Hare WC, et al. An XXY sex-chromosome constitution in a dog with testicular hypoplasia and congenital heart disease. Cytogenetics 1970;9:71–7.
24. Nie GJ, Johnston SD, Hayden DW, et al. Theriogenology question of the month. Azoospermia associated with 79,XXY chromosome complement (canine Klinefelter's syndrome). J Am Vet Med Assoc 1998;212:1545–7.
25. Reimann-Berg N, Escobar HM, Nolte I, et al. Testicular tumor in an XXY dog. Cancer Genet Cytogenet 2008;183:114–6.
26. Centerwall WR, Benirschke K. An animal model for the XXY Klinefelter's syndrome in man: tortoiseshell and calico male cats. Am J Vet Res 1975;36:1275–80.
27. Aksglaede L, Skakkebaek N, Almstrup K, et al. Clinical and biological parameters in 166 boys, adolescents and adults with nonmosaic Klinefelter syndrome: a Copenhagen experience. Acta Paediatr 2011;100:793–806.
28. Smith FW, Buoen LC, Weber AF, et al. X-chromosomal monosomy (77,X0) in a Doberman Pinscher with gonadal dysgenesis. J Vet Intern Med 1989;3:90–5.
29. Lofstedt RM, Buoen LC, Weber AF, et al. Prolonged proestrus in a bitch with X chromosomal monosomy (77,XO). J Am Vet Med Assoc 1992;200:1104–6.
30. Mayenco Aguirre AM, Padilla JA, Flores JM, et al. Canine gonadal dysgenesis syndrome: a case of mosaicism (77,XO-78,XX). Vet Rec 1999;145:582–4.
31. Goldschmidt B, Paulino FO, Souza LM, et al. Infertility related to X-trisomy in a labrador retriever bitch. Israel J Vet Med 2003;58:123–4.

32. Johnston SD, Buoen LC, Weber AF, et al. X trisomy in an Airedale bitch with ovarian dysplasia and primary anestrus. Theriogenology 1985;24:597–607.
33. O'Connor CL, Schweizer C, Gradil C, et al. Trisomy-X with estrous cycle anomalies in two female dogs. Theriogenology 2011;76:374–80.
34. Switonski M, Godynicki S, Jackowiak H, et al. Brief communication. X trisomy in an infertile bitch: cytogenetic, anatomic, and histologic studies. J Hered 2000;91: 149–50.
35. Malan V, Vekemans M, Turleau C. Chimera and other fertilization errors. Clinl Genet 2006;70:363–73.
36. Schelling C, Pienkowska-Schelling A, Arnold S, et al. A male to female sex-reversed dog with a reciprocal translocation. J Reprod Fert Suppl 2001;57:435–8.
37. Dain AR, Walker RG. Two intersex dogs with mosaicism. J Reprod Fertil 1979;56: 239–42.
38. Weaver AD, Harvey MJ, Munro CD, et al. Phenotypic intersex (female pseudohermaphroditism) in a dachshund dog. Vet Rec 1979;105:230–2.
39. Poth T, Breuer W, Walter B, et al. Disorders of sex development in the dog–Adoption of a new nomenclature and reclassification of reported cases. Anim Reprod Sci 2010;121:197–207.
40. Schlafer DH, Valentine B, Fahnestock G, et al. A case of SRY-positive 38,XY true hermaphroditism (XY sex reversal) in a cat. Vet Pathol Online 2011;48:817–22.
41. Meyers-Wallen VN, Schlafer D, Barr I, et al. Sry-negative XX sex reversal in purebred dogs. Mol Reprod Dev 1999;53:266–73.
42. Meyers Wallen VN, Patterson DF. XX sex reversal in the American cocker spaniel dog: phenotypic expression and inheritance. Hum Genet 1988;80:23–30.
43. Curtis E, Grant R. Masculinization of female pups by progestagens. J Am Vet Med Assoc 1964;144:395–8.
44. Knighton E. Congenital adrenal hyperplasia secondary to 11beta-hydroxylase deficiency in a domestic cat. J Am Vet Med Assoc 2004;225:231, 238–41.
45. Nowacka-Woszuk J, Nizanski W, Klimowicz M, et al. Normal male chromosome complement and a lack of the SRY and SOX9 gene mutations in a male pseudohermaphrodite dog. Anim Reprod Sci 2007;98:371–6.
46. Breshears M, Peters J. Diagnostic exercise: ambiguous genitalia in a fertile, unilaterally cryptorchid male miniature schnauzer dog. Vet Pathol 2011;48:E1.
47. Matsuu A, Hashizume T, Kanda T, et al. A case of persistent mullerian duct syndrome with Sertoli cell tumor and hydrometra in a dog. J Vet Med Sci 2009;71:379–81.
48. Vegter AR, Kooistra HS, Van Sluijs FJ, et al. Persistent Mullerian duct syndrome in a miniature schnauzer dog with signs of feminization and a Sertoli cell tumour. Reprod Dom Anim 2010;45:447–52.
49. Marshall LS, Oehlert ML, Haskins ME, et al. Persistent Müllerian duct syndrome in miniature schnauzers. J Am Vet Med Assoc 1982;181:798–801.
50. Kuiper H, Wagner F, Drgemller C, et al. Persistent Mullerian duct syndrome causing male pseudohermaphroditism in a mixed-breed dog. Vet Rec 2004;155:400–1.
51. Nickel R, Ubbink G, van der Gaag I, et al. Persistent mullerian duct syndrome in the basset hound. Tijdschr Diergeneeskd 1992;117(Suppl 1):31S.
52. Meyers-Wallen VN. CVT Update: Inherited disorders of the reproductive tract in dogs and cats. In: Bonagura J, editor. Current veterinary therapy XIV. Philadelphia: WB Saunders; 2008. p. 1034–9.
53. Pujar S, Meyers Wallen VN. A molecular diagnostic test for persistent Müllerian duct syndrome in miniature schnauzer dogs. Sex Dev 2009;3:326–8.
54. Peter AT, Markwelder D, Asem EK. Phenotypic feminization in a genetic male dog caused by nonfunctional androgen receptors. Theriogenology 1993;40:1093–105.

55. Meyers Wallen VN, Wilson JD, Griffin JE, et al. Testicular feminization in a cat. J Am Vet Med Assoc 1989;195:631–4.
56. Yates D, Hayes G, Heffernan M, et al. Incidence of cryptorchidism in dogs and cats. Vet Rec 2003;152:502–4.
57. Dunn M, Foster W, Goddard K. Cryptorchidism in dogs: a clinical survey. Anim Hosp 1968;4:180–2.
58. Boza S, de Membiela F, Navarro A, et al. What is your diagnosis? J Am Vet Med Assoc 2011;238:37–8.
59. Liao AT, Chu P-Y, Yeh L-S, et al. A 12-year retrospective study of canine testicular tumors. J Vet Med Sci 2009;71:919–23.
60. Birchard S, Nappier M. Cryptorchidism. compendiumcom 2008;30:325–36.
61. Zhao X, Du ZQ, Rothschild MF. An association study of 20 candidate genes with cryptorchidism in Siberian husky dogs. J Anim Breed Genet 2010;127:327–31.

Common Lesions in the Male Reproductive Tract of Cats and Dogs

Robert A. Foster, BVSc, PhD, MACVSc

KEYWORDS

• Male • Reproductive • Pathology • Dog • Cat

This article provides an overview of the lesions of the male genital tract of the dog and cat and covers those common diseases that affect the scrotal contents, including testis and epididymis; the accessory genital glands, especially the prostate; and the penis and prepuce.

The majority of lesions of the male reproductive tract of cats and dogs are reported in dogs, and this is reflected in the number and types of diseases listed here. To write an article with an emphasis on "common" lesions presents a particular challenge as the lesions seen, particularly in dogs, varies from one geographical location to another. Defining *common* is also influenced by the behavior of owners and veterinarians. Some common simple lesions such as lacerations are readily identified, are easily treated, and are often not reported. Dramatic lesions may find their way into reports in the literature and assume an unrealistic importance. This article will attempt to balance simple with dramatic lesions and will start with the penis and prepuce, where lesions are seen more commonly.

Male dogs and cats are frequently neutered, and this removes the potential site for lesions to develop (scrotal contents), prevents development of other regions (estrogen- and testosterone-dependent organs such as the prostate and bulbourethral gland), or reduces behaviors that result in lesions in other anatomical sites (penis and prepuce). There are a series of lesions or complications that arise from such surgery and some are listed with the various anatomical sites.

The overall number of potential diseases of the reproductive tract is large and many are obvious and self-explanatory. Readers are advised to examine one or more of the classic textbooks or websites on the subject[1–6] if they find a disease that is not described here.

Much of the material used in this article is found on The Veterinary Reproductive Pathology Website (www.uoguelph.ca/~rfoster/repropath/repro.htm), published by the author.

The author has nothing to disclose.

Department of Pathobiology, Ontario Veterinary College, University of Guelph, 50 Stone Road, Guelph, Ontario, N1G 2W1 Canada
E-mail address: rfoster@uoguelph.ca

Vet Clin Small Anim 42 (2012) 527–545
doi:10.1016/j.cvsm.2012.01.007 vetsmall.theclinics.com

COMMON LESIONS OF THE PENIS AND PREPUCE

The dog and the cat have unique anatomical arrangements of their penis and prepuce. Inflammation of the intrapreputial component of the dog penis is balanitis because it is all part of the head of the penis.[5,6] Inflammation of the intrapreputial component of the feline penis is phallitis because it includes both the head and a portion of the shaft of the penis. The bulbs of the penis in dogs, which swell during erection and form the characteristic bulges on each side, are part of the head of the penis. Some owners, unaware of this unique anatomical feature, consider their presence a "lesion." The prepuce of the dog can be pendulous and expose its contents to foreign objects such as sand. In the cat, the testosterone-dependent barbs are structures that can trap hair and fibers. Many people are unaware that prepubital animals have fusion of the surface of the penis and the internal surface of the prepuce: this is normal, but the exact time of separation is unknown. Failure of adequate separation leads to retained folds of tissue (balanopreputial folds, of which a persistent frenulum is one).[5]

Dog

Posthitis

Non-specific balanoposthitis, or more commonly termed posthitis, occurs in virtually every dog at some stage in his life and usually not long after puberty due to alterations to local innate and adaptive immunity.[4,5] This is a mild and usually clinically insignificant lesion that owners identify as a small amount of purulent discharge from the orifice of the prepuce. Most have normal intrapreputial tissues. Some dogs will have mild hyperemia and in some instances there will be 1- to 2-mm lymphoid nodules within the preputial epithelium.[4]

Canine transmissible venereal tumor

Canine transmissible venereal tumor (CTVT) is a very common lesion in some parts of the world but occurs sporadically elsewhere in animals that travel to areas with a high prevalence of the disease.[7–10] CTVT is a transmissible tumor where neoplastic round cells are transferred from one host to the next. Molecular techniques identify that neoplasms from different continents and collected decades apart are clonal, and while there are 2 subtypes, they have a common origin.[11] The DNA of the CTVT is closely related to DNA of wolves and East Asian dog breeds. The lesions of transmissible venereal tumors are exophytic multinodular proliferations in the preputial cavity, often attached to the junction between the inner sheath of the prepuce and penile epithelium. The size can vary considerably from small to large fungating masses that cause preputial swellings (**Fig. 1**). These tend to be friable, ulcerated, and bleed. Diagnosis of CTVT is by histologic evaluation and differentiation from other round cell tumors.

Paraphimosis, phimosis, and priapism

Paraphimosis is protrusion of the nonerect penis with an inability to retract the penis back into the prepuce. Many cases are idiopathic[12] and likely related to an abnormality with the preputial muscles.[13] Reasons for paraphimosis in the dog include a small preputial orifice, shortened prepuce, weakened preputial muscles, and trauma. The penis that cannot be retracted dries, becomes traumatized, and may swell with edema. It could eventually become completely necrotic from venous infarction secondary to strangulation and venous obstruction.

Priapism is persistent erection of the penis without sexual stimulation. Some definitions include a 4-hour time period. Persistently erect penises become traumatized, dry, or

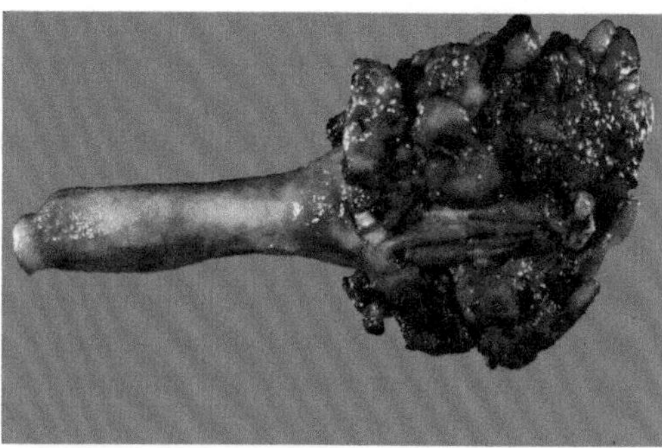

Fig. 1. Canine transmissible venereal tumor, prepuce, dog. Multinodular hemorrhagic masses on the penis at the preputial junction. (*Courtesy of* Department of Pathobiology, Ontario Veterinary College, University of Guelph.)

undergo necrosis. Little is reported about the pathogenesis, but many have spinal lesions that interfere with nervous control of the erection process.[14,15] There are many similarities between priapism and paraphimosis and separating the 2 can be challenging. Priapism develops from trauma, neoplasia, inflammation, or vascular anomaly, or it is idiopathic and "primary."

Phimosis is the inability to extrude the penis. Stenosis of the orifice of the prepuce is the most common cause. This stenosis can be congenital[16] or acquired. It is seldom reported, primarily because it is usually a secondary problem. It is usually impossible to extrude the penis of a prepubertal animal as the penile epithelium is fused to the internal preputial sheath until sometime up until puberty: this is not true phimosis! Phimosis prevents mating, and it also may lead to urine scalding of the prepuce and posthitis. Severe cases have urinary obstruction.

Preputial foreign body

The presence of foreign material within the preputial cavity usually incites a much more florid inflammatory reaction than the typical nonspecific posthitis.[2] Hemorrhage from the prepuce is often an indicator but a more voluminous purulent discharge can occur. The foreign material lacerates the penile mucosa and causes inflammation. Once the foreign body is removed, healing occurs as elsewhere, with regeneration or granulation.

Penile and preputial trauma and ulceration

Ulceration of the penis or prepuce and laceration[2] probably has a similar origin. Affected dogs develop an erect penis that is subsequently traumatized, have foreign material within the prepuce, "tie" with a bitch in a less than ideal situation such as through a wire fence, are forced apart by owners, or develop necrosis of the epithelium during masturbation. The penis and prepuce are traumatized in traffic accidents. Healing with granulation occurs as elsewhere. Adhesions between the penis and prepuce develop only rarely. Polypoid hyperplasia, mucosal tags, and granulation can subsequently develop. These structures are more prone to subsequent trauma. Their presence is usually recognized following hemorrhage from the prepuce. Tags are readily removed without complications.

Penile papilloma

A squamous papilloma is when there is papillary hyperplasia of the epithelium of the penis or prepuce that is supported by a connective-tissue stroma. These papillomas vary in size. No viral cytopathic affect is evident and there is no evidence of direct viral involvement.[17] They arise spontaneously or from local trauma or irritation.

Viral papillomas occur on the penis or preputial mucosa of dogs and they are indistinguishable clinically from nonviral squamous papillomas or even from tags, hyperplastic polyps, or exuberant granulation tissue. These can develop into squamous cell carcinomas; this is a rare occurrence. They are caused by canine papilloma virus and begin with a plaquelike appearance or are raised papillomatous lesions. The appearance of dysplastic and neoplastic cells within the epithelium (in situ carcinoma) and then squamous cell carcinoma suggests progression from one to the other. Their appearance is identical to papillomas elsewhere. They presumably develop from previously injured tissue, as papillomaviruses usually require proliferative epithelium to initiate infection. Histopathology is required to confirm the diagnosis.

Fracture of the os penis

Fracture of the os penis is a well-recognized condition that occurs with local trauma. Pathologic fracture secondary to neoplasia of the os penis is much rarer.

Cat

There are no primary diseases of the penis and prepuce of the cat that could be regarded as "common." The urethra of the penis is a frequent site for sabulous uroliths to lodge. When a urolith does lodge in this location, it can result in penile urethral necrosis and imbibition of urine. The manipulation and insertion of a urethral catheter cause local trauma and erosion of the epithelium of the urethra. Adjacent hemorrhage and edema will further obstruct urethral flow. The development of complete penile necrosis, as occurs in other species, is very unusual.

Many of the diseases seen in other species are recorded in cats but mostly as individual case reports. Priapism, paraphimosis, phimosis, phalopreputial bands including persistent frenulum, constricting band of hair, and local inflammatory polyps are all recorded.[1–6] Of these, there are more reports of phimosis than any others. The cause of phimosis is unknown in most cases and some are congenital.

COMMON LESIONS OF THE ACCESSORY GENITAL GLANDS

There is much written about diseases of the only accessory gland of the dog: the prostate. This is in stark contrast to the cat, where lesions of the prostate and bulbourethral gland are discussed in individual case reports. While it is not the purpose of this article to recapitulate all of the information about the various prostatic diseases of the dog, the most clinically relevant ones will be indicated.

Dog

The similarity of diseases of the prostate of dogs to that of humans has led to an enormous number of studies into the lesions of the canine prostate. Many authors provide an overview of prostate diseases.[18–24]

Prostatic atrophy/hypoplasia

The castration of dogs at a young age removes the trophic endocrine factors, estrogen and testosterone, necessary for prostatic development. This, in effect, induces prostatic hypoplasia. In a similar way, castration causes atrophy. While in the strictest sense this represents a lesion, neither are clinically relevant except as a method of prevention of disease.

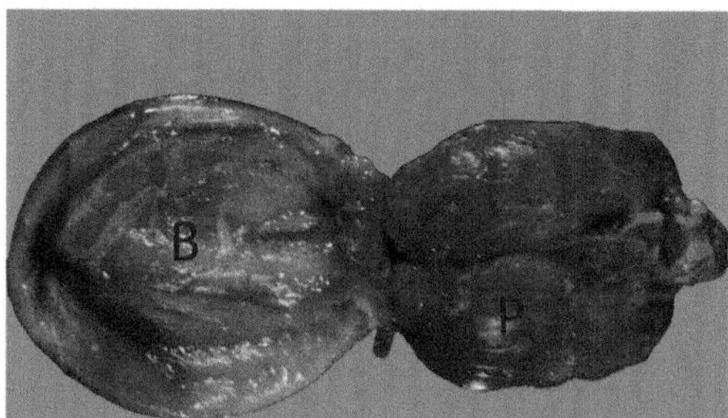

Fig. 2. Prostatic hyperplasia, prostate, dog. Both lobes of the prostate (P) are larger than normal and symmetric with a smooth surface. Bladder (B) is on the left (*Courtesy of* Dr R. Foster, Department of Pathobiology, Ontario Veterinary College, University of Guelph.)

Prostatic hyperplasia/hypertrophy

Canine prostates undergo progressive changes with age. A prepubertal dog has a very small prostate, and with puberty, it increases in size to "normal." About 63% of dogs develop progressive enlargement of the prostate with age after puberty.[22] The enlargement of the prostate with age is difficult to justify as a lesion, and it is common for such a change to be called "benign prostatic hyperplasia" to match the human condition. Some dogs show clinical signs with prostatic enlargement and this has been termed "complicated hyperplasia." When the size of the prostate gland becomes large enough to cause clinical signs, there is fecal obstruction rather than urinary obstruction (as occurs in humans). The hyperplastic prostate is uniformly enlarged. It typically has a smooth capsular surface and the parenchyma is uniform (**Fig. 2**).

Prostatic squamous metaplasia

Squamous metaplasia occurs when the columnar glandular epithelium becomes stratified squamous in type. The mechanism for the development of squamous epithelium involves the production of keratins by the basal cells. The most dramatic forms of squamous metaplasia occur with exposure to estrogens or in feminizing syndromes. Irritation (from inflammation) will also result in squamous metaplasia, but this is a subtle change and not as dramatic as with exposure to estrogens.[25] The prostate can be variably affected so that no abnormalities may be detected grossly. The most severely affected gland will be larger and have multifocal pinpoint to miliary foci of white pasty material. Fibrosis can be dramatic, also.

Prostatitis and prostatic abscess

Inflammation of the prostate, prostatitis, is a common finding even in asymptomatic dogs.[26] Many dogs have foci of inflammatory cells in the interstitial tissues,[27] suggesting that subclinical infection is common. It also occurs in canine brucellosis,[27] which is discussed in detail in an article elsewhere in this issue. Dogs neutered in puppyhood do not develop prostatitis.

Prostatitis occurs by ascending infection—organisms travel from the penis and prepuce via the urethra to the prostate. Hematogenous spread and localization in the prostate are probably the way that *Brucella canis* reaches the prostate, but infection from epididymitis is also possible. There is also the theoretical possibility of infection of the prostate from the bladder and urine.

Once bacteria infect the prostate, they grow within the lumen of the glands, and either elicit an inflammatory response only, invade, or produce endotoxins or

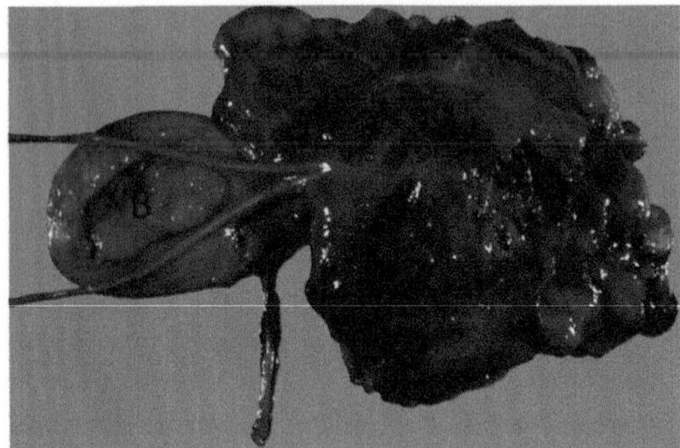

Fig. 3. Prostatitis, prostate, dog. The periprostatic tissues are expanded with edema and hemorrhage so that the prostate is no longer visible. Bladder (B) is on the left. (*Courtesy of* Dr R. Foster, Department of Pathobiology, Ontario Veterinary College, University of Guelph.)

exotoxins. It is likely that ascending infection will have an acute intra-acinar or glandular phase and later a chronic interstitial phase. Bacteria within the lumen of the glands will likely not be recognized by the body, at least not initially.

Acute severe prostatitis is a painful condition that is accompanied by systemic illness. Such cases will have edema and hemorrhage of the prostatic and periprostatic tissues (**Fig. 3**). It is difficult to determine the outline of the prostate because of this acute inflammatory response. When the inflammatory response is suppurative, the prostate will be uniformly enlarged and pus can be expressed when pressure is applied to the prostate. Abscessation of the prostate is one outcome of prostatitis. Prostatic abscess, a cavity with pus (**Fig. 4**), probably develops in a prostatic cyst that develops from prostatic hyperplasia. Paraprostatic pseudocysts are sites for the development of "prostatic abscesses," although these should be called paraprostatic abscesses.

Carcinoma of the prostate

Prostatic carcinoma is a term with several meanings. The convention is that carcinomas of the prostate are adenocarcinoma (from the prostate glandular tissue), and although this

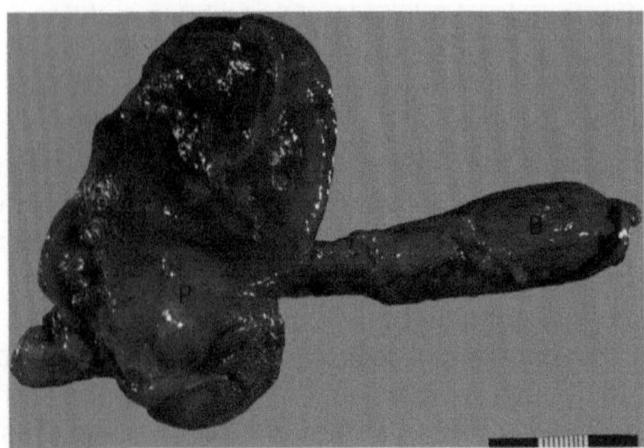

Fig. 4. Prostatic cyst and abscess, and prostatic hypertrophy, prostate, dog. There is a 15-cm cystic structure (C) attached to and extending from the hyperplastic prostate (P). This structure contained pus. The urinary bladder (B) is on the right. (*Courtesy of* Dr R. Foster, Department of Pathobiology, Ontario Veterinary College, University of Guelph.)

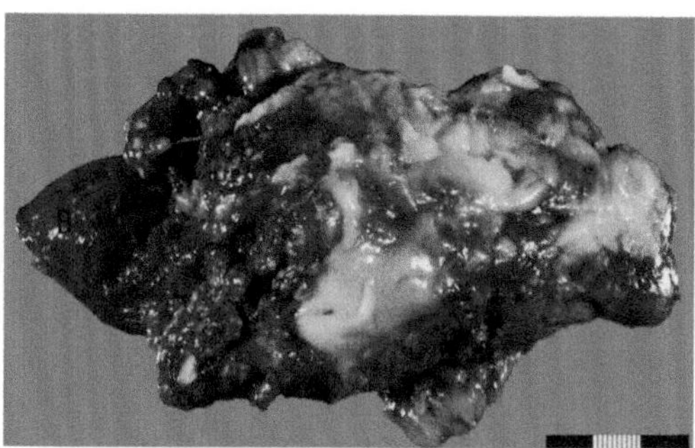

Fig. 5. Carcinoma of the prostate, prostate, dog. The normal prostate is obliterated by infiltrative nodules and fibrosis of a carcinoma. The neoplastic tissue filled the pelvis and infiltrated the intrapelvic tissues. The bladder (B) on the left is is partially obscured by neoplastic tissue. (*Courtesy of* Dr R. Foster, Department of Pathobiology, Ontario Veterinary College, University of Guelph.)

is reasonable in humans, it is not necessarily the case in dogs. There are several types of carcinoma in dogs, including adenocarcinoma (presumably from the glands), transitional cell carcinoma (from the prostatic ducts), mixed carcinomas, and squamous cell carcinomas. There is disagreement as to which is the most common and this is because subclassifying carcinomas is subjective. Prognostically, there is little difference. Virtually every dog develops metastasis,[28] but it is usually the local clinical disease with urinary obstruction and/or incontinence that limits survival. Carcinoma of the prostate occurs in sexually intact and neutered dogs, and there is little difference in prevalence between them,[29] although Teske and colleagues[30] found an increased risk in castrated dogs.

Prostates with neoplasia are highly variable in their appearance. Some, particularly those in neutered dogs, have very little change. Slight enlargement may be the only change. There is usually a central cavity with a fibrous wall, or focal areas of necrosis. At the other extreme is when the prostate is dramatically enlarged, greater than 20 cm in diameter and multinodular, asymmetrical, and with adhesions to the surrounding tissues (**Fig. 5**).

Prostatic and paraprostatic cysts

There are many cysts that develop within and around the prostate. Those around the prostate are grouped as paraprostatic cysts and those within the prostate are called prostatic cysts. Prostatic cysts occurs secondary to prostatic hyperplasia. During age-associated prostatic hyperplasia in intact male dogs, there is variable distension of prostatic acini to form cystic structures. Some of these distended lumens are large enough to be classified as cysts, and some are several centimeters in diameter and give these prostates a polycystic appearance. Some can become infected and become abscesses.

Cat

The cat has 2 accessory genital glands: the prostate and bulbourethral glands. While they are uncommon, prostatic carcinoma, paraprostatic cysts, prostatic abscess, and prostatic squamous metaplasia are reported.[2,4] These are essentially synonymous with the related disease in the dog so readers should refer to the appropriate sections. The bulbourethral gland is well known to surgeons as a reference point for perineal urethrostomy in cats. It is affected by inflammatory disease, as is the prostate. Cystitis and urethritis extend to both the prostate and bulbourethral glands.

COMMON LESIONS OF THE SCROTAL CONTENTS

The scrotum is a sac with an outer layer of skin, a middle layer of connective tissue and the dartos muscle, and an inner lining of serosa identical to peritoneum. The skin responds as does skin over the rest of the body, although in dogs it is mostly devoid of hair. This latter anatomical feature exposes the scrotal skin to contact with irritant agents and to contact dermatitis, including drug reactions and allergic/hypersensitivity reactions.[31,32] The vaginal tunics respond like peritoneum and other serosal surfaces.

Dog

Vaginal tunics, testicular capsule, and peritesticular tissues

The tunics are continuous with the peritoneum, so they are affected by the same diseases as the abdominal cavity. Disease of the tunics can originate from diseases of the abdomen or from the scrotal sac itself. Hematocele is an accumulation of blood within the cavity of the vaginal tunics. Local trauma is the most likely cause, but any disease or condition resulting in hemorrhage can be responsible. Hydrocele is an accumulation of ascitic fluid within the cavity of the vaginal tunic. It will form for all the same reasons as ascites. Hydrocele with fluid restricted to the scrotum is seen secondary to conditions that obstruct lymphatic or venous outflow.[33]

Scrotal (inguinal) hernia is herniation of abdominal contents through the inguinal ring and causes a swelling or mass in the region of the spermatic cord (pampiniform plexus, deferent duct, and cremaster muscle). This occurs as a result of trauma (such as a motor vehicle accident) or it is a spontaneous event.[34] Hernias can occlude vessels of the spermatic cord and cause edema, hydrocele, and/or venous infarction of the testis.

Periorchitis is inflammation around the testis, and it most commonly arises from epididymitis (see later). It can also arise from extension of peritonitis and from penetrating injury to the scrotum. The dependent nature of the scrotal sac means that exudates remain in the sac. Organization and fibrosis of exudates and granulation tissue lead to fibrous adhesions and subsequent testicular atrophy from reduced thermoregulation and pressure.

Testicular disease

Testicular neoplasia

Testicular neoplasia in dogs is very common.[35] Primary testicular neoplasms include sex cord/stroma tumors (interstitial cell tumors, Sertoli cell tumors), germ cell tumors (seminoma, teratoma), and epithelial tumors (rete adenoma and carcinoma).[36] The vast majority are benign; metastatic tumors are rare and unfortunately have no distinguishing feature apart from the presence of metastasis. Neoplasms of dogs may be accompanied by hormonal changes and feminization—especially the Sertoli cell tumor and occasionally the interstitial cell tumor. These same tumors are particularly seen in cryptorchid testes.

Sex cord—stromal (gonadostromal) tumors

Neoplasms with a phenotype resembling the cells that originate from stroma or sex cords of the primitive gonad include the interstitial cell tumor and Sertoli cell tumor. Interstitial (Leydig) cell tumors are almost all well-differentiated tumors and they are almost always benign; while there are no published reports of metastatic interstitial cell tumors, there are anecdotal accounts of them. Interstitial tumors may be hormonally active with either androgenic or estrogenic effects.[37,38] There is no apparent association between cryptorchidism and the development of interstitial cell

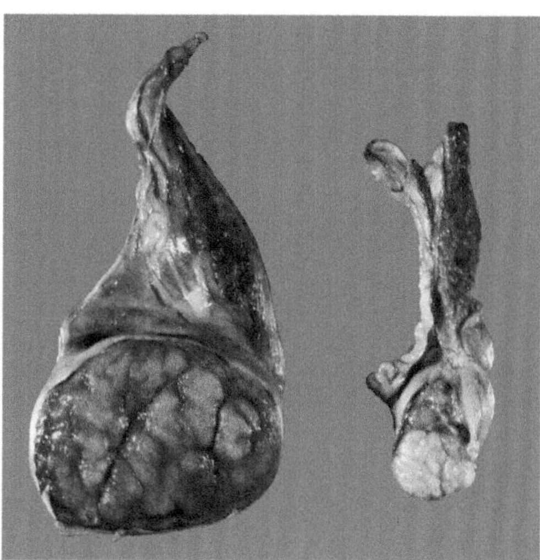

Fig. 6. Bilateral Sertoli cell tumors and cryptorchidism, testis, dog. Both cryptorchid testes are enlarged by Sertoli cell tumors that are white, septate, and very firm and tough. Testicular tissue is no longer visible. (*Courtesy of* Dr R. Foster, Department of Pathobiology, Ontario Veterinary College, University of Guelph.)

tumors. Interstitial cell tumors are well circumscribed and expansile and noninvasive neoplasms that have a tan color. The presence of many vascular channels and, in some, lakes of blood or hemorrhage means they may have large red to black regions throughout. Many are incidental lesions discovered when the testis is routinely cut at surgery or necropsy. Some are large enough to cause testicular enlargement.

Sertoli cell tumors are one of the most common and well known testicular tumors, especially because of their propensity to induce a feminization syndrome.[39] The feminizing effects of some Sertoli cell tumors include the presence of gynecomastia, attraction of affected dogs to other male dogs, alopecia, and hyperpigmentation, and testicular atrophy. They arise especially in cryptorchid testes and those in the abdomen are more likely to be affected. Metastatic disease has been found, but it is rare. Metastasis, when present, is often to the spermatic cord but some are to the local lymph node or beyond.[34,39] Sertoli cell tumors are mostly found when there is hormonal secretion or testicular and/or scrotal enlargement. There is a suggestion that the secondary effects are related to the size of the neoplasm, and as such, cryptorchid testes that achieve a large size are more likely to have feminization effects. Dogs can develop prostatic disease from prostatic hyperplasia and from squamous metaplasia. There may be pancytopenia that is poorly responsive and bleeding tendencies. They are usually expansile and well-demarcated tumors that are solid and some contain cystic spaces. The neoplasm is usually white, but some are red or red-brown. They are often hard to cut and do not appreciably bulge on cut section. Beams or trabeculae of fibrous tissue are usually prominent and abundant (**Fig. 6**).

Germ cell tumors

Germ cell tumors of the canine testis are of 2 types: those cells with a phenotype of spermatogonia and spermatocytes (called seminomas) and those that display pluripotency, being able to differentiate to any tissue in the body including ectoderm,

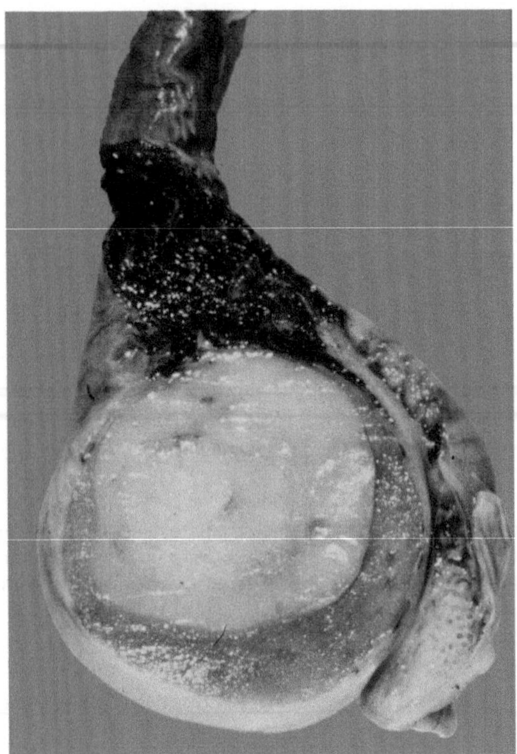

Fig. 7. Seminoma, testis, dog. There is a well-circumscribed white homogeneous neoplasm in the testis. Residual testis is brown and atrophic, and compressed to the periphery of the seminoma. (*Courtesy of* Dr R. Foster, Department of Pathobiology, Ontario Veterinary College, University of Guelph.)

mesoderm, and endoderm (called teratomas). Seminomas are very common in dogs; they are a more primitive and poorly differentiated type of neoplasm. Teratomas are rare.[2,35] Seminomas cause testicular enlargement as the main clinical sign. Seminomas have 2 main patterns: an intratubular type that is often microscopic and found incidentally and a diffuse type. It is assumed that they begin as intratubular neoplasms that expand to form the diffuse type. Older dogs are more likely to be affected, and there is an increased prevalence in cryptorchid testis, especially those that are inguinally retained. Testicular seminomas have a characteristic appearance in the dog. They are usually found when they cause testicular enlargement, so they form an intratesticular mass. This mass is well circumscribed, white, and homogeneous (**Fig. 7**) and rarely have obvious necrosis or hemorrhage when small. There is no obvious septation, although some can be multilobular. They typically are soft and bulge on cut section. Intratubular seminoma is a histologic diagnosis and is usually incidental. The majority of seminomas are benign and metastatic seminomas are very rare. This is despite their histologic appearance, which, based on first principles, have features of malignancy. When they do metastasize, they spread to the spermatic cord and beyond.

Extratesticular testicular tumors in previously neutered dogs

Primary testicular tumors may be found in previously neutered dogs.[40] This is an underrecognized disease. Sertoli cell tumors are the most common but occasional interstitial cell tumors occur. Dogs are typically castrated as juveniles and develop neoplasia later in life, either in the spermatic cord, at the site of the prescrotal incision, or in the scrotal skin. It is assumed that the neoplasms arose from testicular tissue implanted after the testis is inadvertently incised during castration. Most of the neoplasms were small and about 1.5 cm in diameter. Their appearance, apart from their location, is identical to their intratesticular counterpart. Excision is curative.

Small or missing testes

1. Previous surgical removal: An absence of a scrotal testis means that the testis was previously removed, or it is retained or cryptorchid. When there is previous surgical removal, the end of the deferent duct can be found, is well developed, and is of a size commensurate with the size of the duct at the age of castration or removal. No epididymal tissues or embryonic remnants should be present.
2. Cryptorchidism (retained testes): Cryptorchid or retained testes are those that did not complete migration from the retroperitoneal area near the kidney into the scrotum. It is a disorder of sexual development (XY *SRY*+ testicular DSD). Retained testes are seen sporadically as an isolated event and may have a hereditary basis or they are seen in dogs with other disorders of sexual development—for example, miniature schnauzers with persistent Müllerian duct syndrome (PMDS) often have retained testes.[41] There are many breeds of dogs with an increased risk and for which the disease is familial. The heritability appears to be autosomal recessive.

   Most cryptorchids are unilateral and right sided, with inguinal retention being more common than intra-abdominal retention.[42–44] Cryptorchid testes are hypoplastic and as such are the same size as prepubertal testes, at least initially. They will become degenerate and therefore atrophy and become even smaller with time. The size of the epididymis is as expected for a prepubertal epididymis. On occasion, the testis suffers a severe process where it dies from what is assumed to be a vascular event. Torsion of the retained testis can occur and both testis and epididymis will be affected. There are several complications of cryptorchidism including testicular neoplasia, especially Sertoli cell (see **Fig. 6**) tumor and seminoma,[45–47] torsion of the testis, testicular atrophy, and complications of castration.
3. Testicular hypoplasia: Testicular hypoplasia is where the testis does not develop to its normal size.[2,4,5] It is always accompanied by a failure of the epididymis to acquire its normal size. Most cases of hypoplasia are because of cryptorchidism, and primary hypoplasia is limited to those situations where the testis has descended normally. Hypoplasia is almost always seen as a failure of the prepubertal testis to enlarge, but there may be cases where even the prepubertal testis is smaller than normal. Hypoplasia is best diagnosed clinically by identifying that the testis has not increased in size from puberty, but this is seldom monitored in dogs and so the presence of a small testis could mean either hypoplasia or atrophy. Atrophy is an acquired condition, but hypoplasia is potentially a genetic and heritable condition. Hypoplasia may accompany chromosomal abnormalities (chromosomal DSD). The majority of affected testes have reduced spermatogenesis and arrest of spermatogenesis at any stage. The whole testis could be involved or just some of seminiferous tubules. Hypoplasia is variable in its degree from barely detectable to extreme. The testis has a normal shape and tone but is smaller than it should be.[47]
4. Testicular atrophy–degeneration: Testicular atrophy is when the testis becomes smaller in size. It is a clinical or macroscopic term, whereas the corresponding microscopic change is degeneration. It is difficult to differentiate atrophy from

hypoplasia, and knowledge that the testis has became smaller is helpful. The causes of testicular atrophy–degeneration are legion. Some of the known causes are heat including high environmental temperature, fever, epididymitis and orchitis, scrotal dermatitis, scrotal edema, and periorchitis; radiation (for cancer therapy); poor health and debility; advancing age; hormones, including estrogen and Sertoli cell tumors; drugs; chemotherapy; systemic inflammatory diseases; and situations of oxidative stress. Mild degenerative changes occur in dogs with aging. Drugs known to affect infertility include steroidal compounds (methyltestosterone, estradiol, diethylstilbestrol, KABI1774, betamethasone, prednisolone); contraceptive compounds; tamoxifen citrate; gossypol; chemotherapeutic agents, busulfan, chlorambucil, cisplatin, cyclophosphamide, methotrexate, vincristine; and miscellaneous drugs, anticholinergics, barbiturates, chlorpromazine, diazepam, digoxin, levodopa, phenytoin, primidone, propranolol, thiazine diuretics, and verapamil.[48]

In mild forms of atrophy, the testis loses its tone. With increased severity, the testis becomes smaller and firmer as fibrosis develops. An atrophic testis has a normally sized epididymis so the proportions change with increased severity. When there is advanced atrophy, the capsule of the testis is white and thick and the testicular vessels are less obvious or missing. On cut section, an atrophic testis may be red-brown (**Fig. 7**) or could contain bands of or diffuse white areas of fibrosis. Mineralization can also occur, often beginning at the mediastinum and extending outward.

Larger testes

Testicular dissymmetry is a common clinical presentation. Because neoplasia is so common, the natural assumption is that the larger testis is abnormal and neoplastic. The other possibility is unilateral testicular atrophy. A combination can occur with one being smaller, and the other larger. Neoplasia is a common cause of testicular enlargement and is described earlier. Some testicular neoplasms cause testicular atrophy of the contralateral testis, so dissymmetry is exaggerated. Testicular hypertrophy is seldom considered, though. This enlargement is not dramatic. The basis is greater stimulation of interstitial endocrine cells and Sertoli cells by luteinizing hormone and follicle-stimulating hormone that are not sufficiently inhibited in a negative feedback system. Compensatory hypertrophy occurs to its maximal (125%) with unilateral castration or even testicular retention from birth.[49] Adult unilateral castration does not apparently result in hypertrophy.[50] The hypertrophic testis is more bulbous than normal.

Orchitis

From a lesion point of view, orchitis is inflammation of the testis. Clinically though, orchitis is used to indicate any disease of the scrotal contents, including periorchitis, epididymitis, and orchitis itself. Orchitis is, in general, uncommon. Orchitis is identified as a swollen painful testis and is usually accompanied by epididymitis and/or periorchitis. This is so much so that they are combined as epididymo-orchitis. Microscopic orchitis either is an incidental finding when the testis is examined microscopically for another condition or is reported after biopsy of the testis to determine the cause of azoospermia. There is little published about this latter type of orchitis. It is a lymphocytic disease with the seminiferous tubule being the target. The clinical "signs" are azoospermia with or without testicular atrophy.

Testicular torsion and death

Testicular death (necrosis) is when regions of or the whole testis dies. The blood flow to the testis is via a tortuous testicular artery that is part of the pampiniform plexus.

By the time the blood reaches the testis, it is barely pulsate and has a lower pressure than normal arterial pressure. A slight change in flow will result in ischemia. Death of the testis is particularly seen in retained (or cryptorchid) testes and is assumed to occur because of vascular compromise. Torsion of the spermatic cord of a fully descended testis is virtually impossible. It is usually seen in cryptorchid testes as there is sufficient laxity of the gubernaculum to allow the twist. In a normally descended testis, the attachment of the vaginal tunic precludes a twist from occurring.

Torsion will produce venous infarction, with both testis and epididymis becoming hemorrhagic. Death of the testis is an expected sequela. When only the testis and not the epididymis is dead, some vascular event apart from torsion should be invoked. Edema, inflammation, or anything reducing testicular arterial pressure (as occurs in anesthesia), increasing venous pressure, or slowing blood flow could induce necrosis. Anything that increases intratesticular pressure above testicular venous pressure will obstruct blood flow. Testicular torsion may be identified clinically as an "acute abdomen" in a cryptorchid dog. Many are silent and there are remains of a small degenerate gonad. Torsion is more likely to occur in those testes that contain testicular tumors.[51] A necrotic testis has a black or brown-black color, and the cut surface is often dry.

Testicular rupture

Pressure sufficient to overcome the ability of the capsule of the testis to contain the testicular parenchyma will result in rupture. Bite wounds can produce severe injuries including penetrating and crushing wounds. Local blunt force trauma could do this, but it is a rare event. The outcome of testicular rupture is 2-fold. There will be severe trauma and the formation of a hematocele, and inflammation will occur. Rupture and exposure of the germinal cells, that are outside the blood testis barrier, as well as altering the environment and therefore the anti-inflammatory properties of the testis, will induce a foreign body–type reaction (granulomatous), and immune mechanisms will be mediated to induce a further reaction. This is particularly the case in postpubertal animals.

Epididymal disease

Dog

Infectious epididymitis is the most common disease[2,4,5] but is not well studied in dogs. The other 2 important diseases are often missed; they are spermatic granuloma of the epididymal head and segmental aplasia. The presence of spermatozoa, which are antigenic and which also induce a foreign body granulomatous response, complicates the responses of this organ to injury. Spermatozoa are continuously produced, and any obstruction of the single duct of the epididymis results in increased pressure and the likelihood of rupture. A rupture or perforation of the tube will eventually lead to the formation of a spermatocele, a cavity containing impacted spermatozoa. In severe cases, the spermatozoa will be released into the cavity of the vaginal tunics and cause periorchitis. Spermatic granulomas develop anywhere that spermatozoa are found. Most cases occur because of infectious epididymitis, blind efferent ductules, aberrant epididymal ducts, and adenomyosis of the epididymis.

Infectious epididymitis

Epididymitis is complicated by a combination of response to an inciting agent, if present, and to spermatozoa and seminal fluids. Bacterial infection of the epididymis

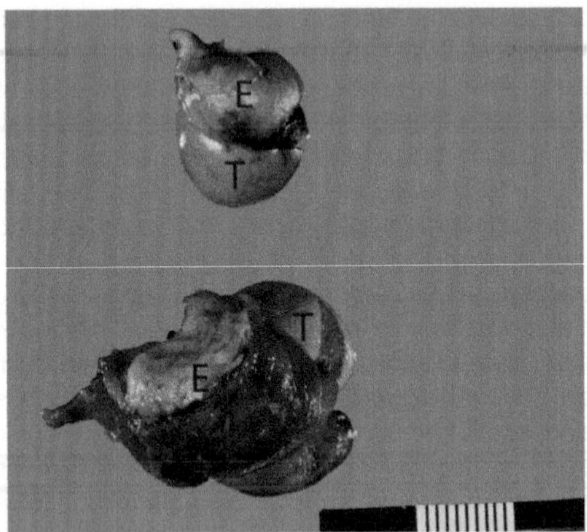

Fig. 8. Unilateral epididymitis, tail of the epididymis, dog. The tail of the epididymis (E) viewed from the ventral surface and attached to the lower testis (T) is much larger than normal (*upper*). The affected epididymis is also red with hemorrhage, and covered with fibrin. (*Courtesy of* Dr R. Foster, Department of Pathobiology, Ontario Veterinary College, University of Guelph.)

is the most common and occurs via 2 main routes: ascending infection from the urethra via the deferent duct and accessory genital glands, or hematogenous spread. Descending infection from the testis and direct penetrating injury are both theoretically possible but much less likely. *Brucella canis* is a traditional and important cause[52,53] and is discussed in an article elsewhere in this issue. Infections with other gram-negative organisms such as *Escherichia coli* are the most common in other areas. The appearance of epididymitis is similar, regardless of the cause.

The lesions of epididymitis usually involve the tail and sometimes the body of the epididymis; the head of the epididymis is seldom involved. This may be bilateral or unilateral, and the severity varies and reflects the degree of damage, including necrosis and vascular changes. In severe acute disease, there is swelling and edema of the tail of the epididymis. Fibrin appears on the surface of the epididymis and the tunics (**Fig. 8**). The scrotum becomes edematous and swollen. The inflammation is neutrophilic and abscesses form. Release of spermatozoa into the tissues adds to this, and the liquid, although resembling pus, becomes part of a spermatic granuloma. Self-trauma of the scrotum, presumably because of pain, can result in ulceration of the scrotum. The testis can also be involved either with a necrotic orchitis or with necrosis. With time, fibrosis becomes the major lesion, and there will be a marked interstitial fibrosis. Adhesion of the parietal to the visceral vaginal tunic is a common occurrence, and the tunics can become markedly thickened with granulation and fibrous tissue.

Spermatic granuloma of the epididymal head

Spermatic granuloma of the epididymal head is a condition that is underrecognized. Many cases of obstructive azoospermia without infectious epididymitis are due to this. It is a congenital condition that usually is only recognized (if at all) at puberty when spermatozoa are produced. It is the end result of efferent ductules failing to join to the epididymal duct at the region of the head of the epididymis. At puberty,

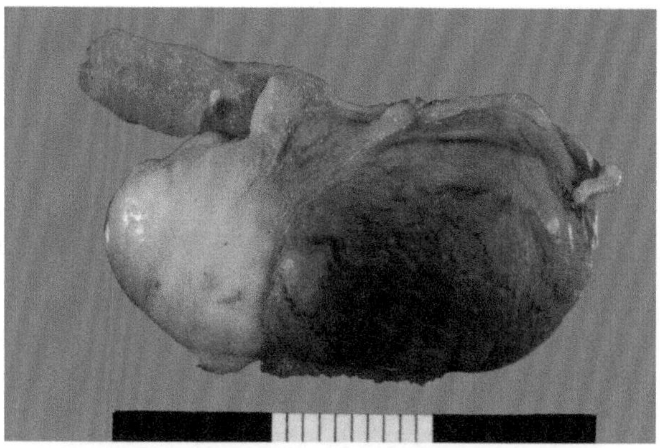

Fig. 9. Spermatic granuloma of the epididymal head, head of the epididymis, dog. The white nodule beneath the pampiniform plexus, and at the cranial pole of the testis is a spermatic granuloma formed from blind-ending efferent ductules. (*Courtesy of* Dr R. Foster, Department of Pathobiology, Ontario Veterinary College, University of Guelph.)

spermatozoa are forced into the blind-ended tubule and form a spermatocele and eventually a spermatic granuloma. It is probably a genetic-hereditary disease.[2] Small lesions are only seen when the region of the efferent ducts and head of the epididymis are examined carefully. A white nodule of several millimeters' diameter up to 1 cm within the tissue is the only finding (**Fig. 9**). Astute practitioners can detect larger examples through scrotal palpation.

Segmental aplasia of the mesonephric duct

Segmental aplasia or lack of development of any part of the mesonephric duct, from which is derived the epididymis and deferent duct, is assumed to be an inherited disease. Only animals with unilateral disease are fertile,[54] and most cases reported are unilateral. Most cases involve the epididymis, but some also have a lack of the deferent duct (**Fig. 10**). As with spermatic granuloma of the epididymal head, this is an underreported disease that is often missed at scrotal palpation. It is commonly missed at castration, too!

Cat

Trauma, bite wounds, and penetrating injury occur to the tail, base of the tail, and perineal regions including the scrotal skin. Any penetrating wound of the scrotum can result in periorchitis. The peritoneal recess that forms the vaginal tunics is susceptible to local infection and inflammation. This inflammation, called periorchitis, is usually fibrinosuppurative and the scrotum becomes distended and painful. Secondary changes to the testis, including testicular necrosis/infarction, can occur. It is usual for testicular atrophy to be found. Differentiation from feline infectious peritonitis (FIP) can be a challenge. Inflammation of the tunics can occur as a complication of castration when there is infection or a reaction to hair. Periorchitis can also occur secondarily to orchitis or epididymitis but this is very rare in cats.

FIP has many different manifestations. Involvement of the peritoneum, although not always found, can involve the peritesticular region and therefore periorchitis (**Fig. 11**). Involvement of the vaginal tunics is sometimes the first indication of the presence of FIP. In most circumstances, the testis is not directly affected although a primary

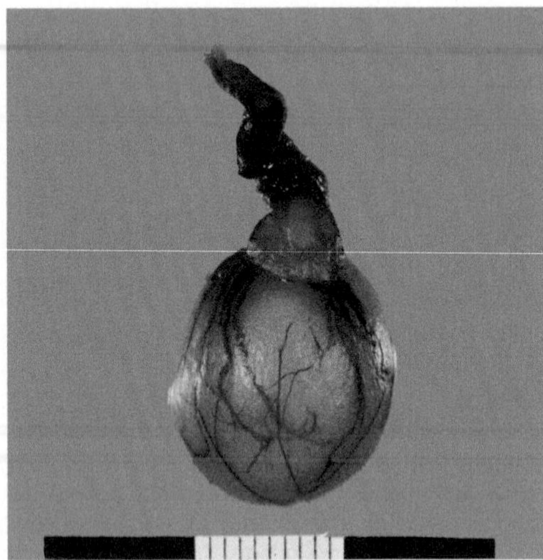

Fig. 10. Segmental aplasia of the mesonephric duct, epididymis, and deferent duct, cat. The head, body, and tail of the epididymis are missing from this testis. (*Courtesy of* Dr R. Foster, Department of Pathobiology, Ontario Veterinary College, University of Guelph.)

orchitis is possible. FIP can be difficult to separate from traumatic/bacterial periorchitis. Lesions of the scrotal skin would not be expected in FIP.

The most common disease of the testis is a failure of testicular descent and is a disorder of sexual development because there is a defect in the transmigration of the testis from its origin near the kidney into the scrotal sac.[55–57] Disorders of sexual development are covered in detail in an article elsewhere in this issue.

SUMMARY

In this overview, common and important diseases of the male reproductive system were discussed with an emphasis on the cause, mechanisms of disease and lesions

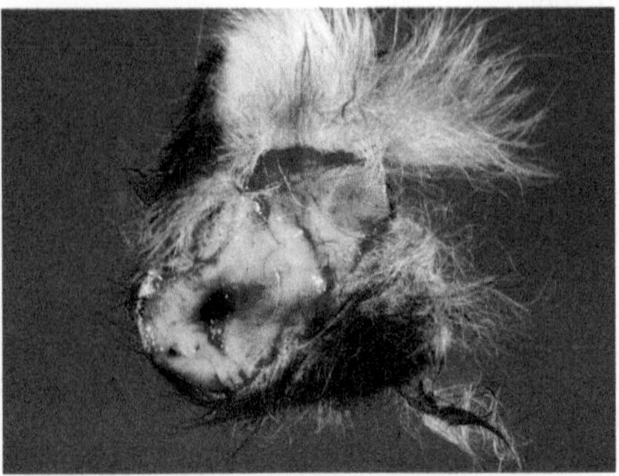

Fig. 11. Feline infectious peritonitis, vaginal tunics of scrotum, cat. The vaginal tunics are 5 mm thick and covered with fibrin and granulomatous inflammation of the effusive form of feline infectious peritonitis of the scrotum. (*Courtesy of* Dr R. Foster, Department of Pathobiology, Ontario Veterinary College, University of Guelph.)

seen. This was done using the approach of identifying region of the reproductive tract, and the basic change particularly whether the organ was smaller or larger than normal. Emphasis is given to those diseases likely to cause infertility and which may be hereditary.

REFERENCES

1. Bloom F. Pathology of the dog and cat: The genitourinary system, with clinical considerations. Evanston (IL): American Veterinary Publications; 1954.
2. McEntee K. Reproductive pathology of domestic mammals. San Diego (CA): Academic Press; 1990.
3. Feldman EC, Nelson RW. Canine and feline endocrinology and reproduction. Philadelphia; Saunders: 2004. p. 953–1004.
4. Foster RA, Ladds PW. The male genital system. In: Maxie G, editor. Jubb, Kennedy & Palmer's pathology of domestic animals, vol. 3. 5th edition. Toronto: A Saunders Ltd; 2007. p. 565–619.
5. Foster RA. Male reproductive system. In: Zachary J, McGavin DM, editors. Pathologic basis of veterinary disease. 5th edition. St Louis: Elsevier Mosby; 2011. p. 1127–52.
6. Foster RA. The veterinary reproductive pathology Website. Available at: www.uoguelph.ca/~rfoster/repropath/repro.htm. Accessed January 27, 2012.
7. Ndiritu CG. Lesions of the canine penis and prepuce. Mod Vet Pract 1979;60:712–5.
8. Cohen D. The transmissible venereal tumor of the dog: a naturally occurring allograft? a review. Israel J Med Sci 1978;14:14–9.
9. Mukaratirwa S, Gruys E. Canine transmissible venereal tumor: cytogenetic origin, immunophenotype, and immunobiology. A review. Vet Q 2003;25:101–11.
10. Mello-Martins MI, Ferreira de Souza F, Gobello C. Canine transmissible venereal tumor: etiology, pathology, diagnosis and treatment. In: Concannon PW, England G, Verstgegen J, et al, editors. Recent advances in small animal reproduction. Available at: www.ivis.org. Accessed January 27, 2012.
11. Murgia C, Pritchard JK, Kim SY, et al. Clonal origin and evolution of a transmissible cancer. Cell 2006;126:477–87.
12. Papazoglou LG. Idiopathic chronic penile protrusion in the dog: a report of six cases. J Small Anim Pract 2001;42:510–3.
13. Chaffee VW, Knecht CD. Canine paraphimosis: sequel to inefficient preputial muscles. Vet Med Small Anim Clin 1975;70:1418–20.
14. Rochat MC. Priapism: a review. Theriogenology 2001;56:713–22.
15. Lavely JA. Priapism in dogs. Top Comp Anim Med 2009;24:49–54.
16. Sarierler M, Kara ME. Congenital stenosis of the preputial orifice in a dog. Vet Rec 1998;143:201.
17. Cornegliani L, Vercelli A, Abramo F. Idiopathic mucosal penile squamous papillomas in dogs. Vet Dermatol 2007;18:439–43.
18. O'Shea JD. Studies on the canine prostate gland, 1: factors influencing its size and weight. J Comp Pathol 1962;72:321–31.
19. Hornbuckle WE, MacCoy DM, Allan GS, et al. Prostatic disease in the dog. Cornell Vet 1978;68(Suppl 7):284–305.
20. Basanti JA, Finco DR. Canine prostatic diseases. Vet Clin North Am Small Anim Pract 1986;16:587–99.
21. Olson PN, Wrigley RH, Thrall MA, et al. Disorders of the canine prostate gland: pathogenesis, diagnosis, and medical therapy. Compend Contin Educ Small Anim 1987;9:613–23.
22. Krawiec DR. Canine prostatic disease. J Am Vet Med Assoc 1994;204:1561–4.

23. Krawiec DR, Helfin D. Study of prostatic disease in dogs: 177 cases (1981–1986). J Am Vet Med Assoc 1992;200:1119–22.
24. Johnston SD, Kamolpatana K, Root-Kustritz MV, et al. Prostatic disorders in the dog. Anim Reprod Sci 2000;60–61:405–15.
25. O'Shea JD. Squamous metaplasia of the canine prostate gland. Res Vet Sci 1963;4: 431–4.
26. Diniz SA, Melo MS, Borges AM, et al. Genital lesions associated with visceral leishmaniasis and shedding of Leishmania sp. in the semen of naturally infected dogs. Vet Pathol 2005;42:650–8.
27. Brennan SJ, Ngeleka M, Philibert HM, et al. Canine brucellosis in a Saskatchewan kennel. Can Vet J 2008;49:703–8.
28. Leav I, Ling GV. Adenocarcinoma of the canine prostate. Cancer 1968;22:1329–45.
29. Bell RW, Klausner JS, Hayden DW, et al. Clinical and pathologic features of prostatic adenocarcinoma in sexually intact and castrated dogs: 31 cases (1970–1987). J Am Vet Med Assoc 1991;199:1623.
30. Teske E, Naan EC, van Dijk EM, et al. Canine prostate carcinoma: epidemiological evidence of an increased risk in castrated dogs. Mol Cell Endocrinol 2002;197:251–5.
31. Cerundolo R, Maiolino P. Cutaneous lesions of the canine scrotum. Vet Dermatol 2002;13:63–76.
32. Trenti D, Carlotti DN, Pin D, et al. Suspected contact scrotal dermatitis in the dog: a retrospective study of 13 cases (1987 to 2003). J Small Anim Pract 2011;52:295–300.
33. McNeil PE, Weaver AD. Massive scrotal swelling in two unusual cases of canine Sertoli cell tumour. Vet Rec 1980;106:144–6.
34. Dorn AS. Spermatic cord occlusion in a dog. J Am Vet Med Assoc 1978;173:81.
35. Kennedy PC, Cullen JM, Edwards JF, et al. Histological classification of tumors of the genital system of domestic animals. World Health Organisation International histological classification of tumors of domestic animals. Washington, DC: Armed Forces Institute of Pathology and American Registry of Pathology; 1998.
36. Peters MAJ, de Long FH, Teerds KJ, et al. Ageing, testicular tumors and pituitary-testis axis in dogs. J Endocrinol 2000;166:153–61.
37. Mischke R, Meurer D, Hoppen H-O, et al. Blood plasma concentrations of estradiol-17B, testosterone and testosterone/oestradiol ratio in dogs with neoplastic and degenerative testicular diseases. Res Vet Sci 2002;73:267–72.
38. Brodey RS, Martin JE. Sertoli cell neoplasms in the dog: the clinicopathological and endocrinological findings in 37 dogs. J Am Vet Med Assoc 1958;133:249–57.
39. Coffin DL, Munson TO, Scully RE. Functional Sertoli cell tumour with metastasis in a dog. J Am Vet Med Assoc 1952;121(908):352–8.
40. Doxsee AL, Yager JA, Best SJ, et al. Extratesticular interstitial and Sertoli cell tumors in previously neutered dogs and cats: a report of 17 cases. Can Vet J 2006;47:763–6.
41. Marshall LS, Oehlert ML, Haskins ME, et al. Persistent mullerian duct syndrome in miniature schnauzers. J Am Vet Med Assoc 1982;181:798–801.
42. Romagnoli SE. Canine cryptorchidism. Vet Clin North Am Small Anim Pract 1991;21: 533–44.
43. Yates D, Hayes G, Heffernan M, et al. Incidence of cryptorchidism in dogs and cats. Vet Rec 2003;152:502–4.
44. Reif JS, Brodey RS. The relationship between cryptorchidism and canine testicular neoplasia. J Am Vet Med Assoc 1969;155:2005–10.
45. Pendergrass TW, Hayes HM. Cryptorchidism and related defects in dogs: epidemiologic comparisons with man. Teratology 1975;12:51–6.

46. Hayes HM, Wilson GP, Pendergrass TW, et al. Canine cryptorchidism and subsequent testicular neoplasia: case control study with epidemiologic update. Teratology 1985;32:51–6.
47. Ortega-Pacheco A, Rodríguez-Buenfil JC, Segura-Correa1 JC, et al. Pathological conditions of the reproductive organs of male stray dogs in the tropics: prevalence, risk factors, morphological findings and testosterone concentrations. Reprod Dom Anim 2006;41:429–37.
48. Freshman JL. Drugs affecting fertility in the male dog. Current veterinary therapy, X, small animal practice. Toronto: WB Saunders, 1989. p. 1225.
49. Tsutsui T, Kurita A, Kirihara N, et al. Testicular compensatory hypertrophy related to hemicastration in prepubertal dogs. J Vet Med Sci 2004;66:1021–5.
50. Taha MA, Noakes DE, Allen WE. Hemicastration and castration in the beagle dog; the effect on libido, plasma testosterone concentrations, seminal characteristics and testicular function. J Sm Anim Pract 1982;23:279–85.
51. Pearson H, Kelly DF. Testicular torsion in the dog: a review of 13 cases. Vet Rec 1975;97:200–4.
52. Barr SC, Eitis BE, Roy AF, et al. Brucella suis biotype 1 infection in a dog. J Am Vet Med Assoc 1986;189:686–7.
53. Wanke MM. (2004) Canine brucellosis. Anim Reprod Sci 2004;82–83:195–207.
54. Olson PN, Schultheiss P, Seim HB. Clinical and laboratory findings associated with actual or suspected azoospermia in dogs: 18 cases (1979). J Am Vet Med Assoc 1992;201:478–4.
55. Millis DL, Hauptman JG, Johnson CA. Cryptorchidism and monorchism in cats: 25 cases (1980–1989). J Am Vet Med Assoc 1992;200:1128–30.
56. Yates D, Hayes G, Heffernan M, et al. Incidence of cryptorchidism in dogs and cats. Vet Rec 2003;152:502–4.
57. Centerwall WR, Benirschke K. An animal model for the XXY Klinefelter's syndrome in man: tortoiseshell and calico male cats. Am J Vet Res 1975;36:1275–80.

Common Lesions in the Female Reproductive Tract of Dogs and Cats

Antonio Ortega-Pacheco, DVM, MVSc, PhD[a,*],
Eduardo Gutiérrez-Blanco, DVM, MSc[a],
Matilde Jiménez-Coello, DVM, MSc, PhD[b]

KEYWORDS

• Bitch • Pathology • Queen • Reproductive

Our knowledge and understanding of female reproductive physiology and endocrinology in dogs and cats have grown exponentially. In turn, this has helped us gain a better understanding of fertility problems in these species that may originate from pathologic changes throughout the reproductive tract. Private practitioners working on small animal species are commonly confronted with lesions in the female reproductive tract. Many of these lesions may be appear at any time during the reproductive life of the patients. In order to avoid unnecessary therapy or treatment delay, it is important for the clinician to quickly recognize and understand the pathology of the most common reproductive lesions to achieve a rapid and effective diagnosis. Epidemiological investigations into small animal reproductive health demonstrate that certain reproductive lesions may occur more frequently in the bitch and queen, so the clinician must be aware of the range of differential diagnosis and the clinical approach. This article gives an overview of the pathology, clinical and therapy signs of the most common lesions that affect the ovaries, uterus, cervix and vagina in the bitch and queen that may be encountered in practice.

COMMON LESIONS IN THE OVARY

Ovarian Remnant Syndrome

Retention of active ovarian tissue, or "remnant ovarian tissue" (ROT), due to improper clamping of the ovarian pedicle during an ovariectomy or ovariohysterectomy (OVH)

The authors have nothing to disclose.

[a] Departamento de Salud Animal y Medicina Preventiva, Universidad Autónoma de Yucatán, Campus de Ciencias Biológicas y Agropecuarias, Km. 15.5 Carretera Mérida-Xmatkuil, AP 4-116 Mérida, Yucatán, México

[b] CA Biomedicina de Enfermedades Infecciosas y Parasitarias, Laboratorio de Biología Celular, Centro de Investigaciones Regionales "Dr. Hideyo Noguchi" Unidad Biomédica, Universidad Autónoma de Yucatán, Av Itzáez No. 490 x C. 59, CP 97000, Mérida, Yucatán, México

* Corresponding author.

E-mail address: opacheco@uady.mx

Vet Clin Small Anim 42 (2012) 547–559
doi:10.1016/j.cvsm.2012.01.011 vetsmall.theclinics.com
0195-5616/12/$ – see front matter

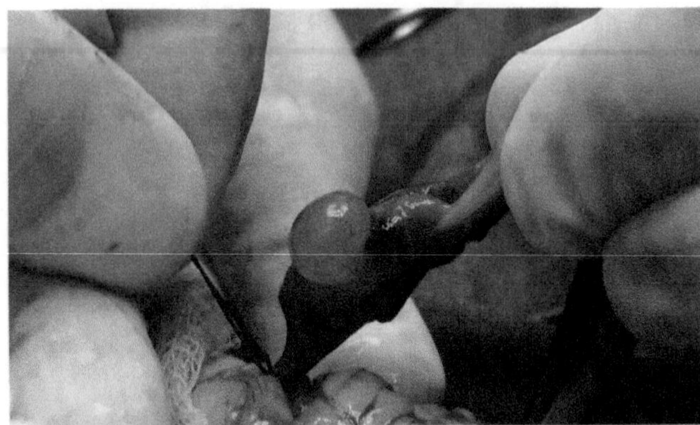

Fig. 1. A 2.2 × 1.8 cm follicular cyst in a queen with persistent estrual activity. (*Courtesy of* Rita López, UADY, School of Veterinary Medicine.)

is an iatrogenic condition commonly seen in the bitch and queen.[1] The presence of an accessory ovary or losing the ovary in the abdomen during surgery can produce similar clinical signs. Under experimental conditions, autografted hemiovaries in the abdominal cavity in dogs have demonstrated good implantation and further ovarian activity.[2]

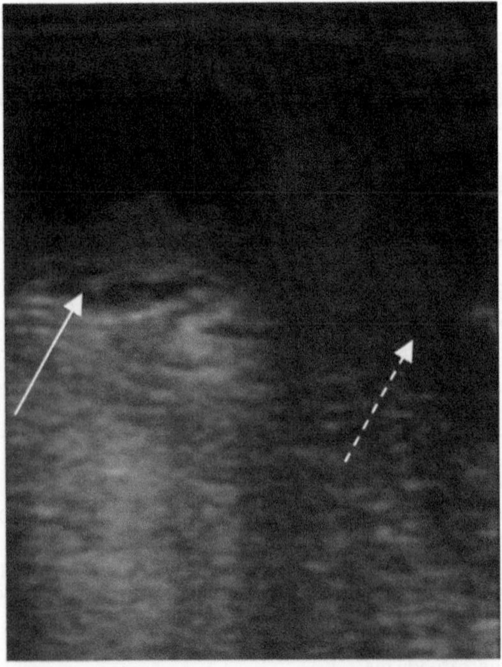

Fig. 2. Ultrasound image of a 2.5-cm follicular cyst in a bitch with history of irregular heats. Ovary (*continuous arrow*) is localized at the caudal pole of the left kidney (*broken arrow*). A process of luteinization can be observed inside the follicle. Small follicles are also present in the ovary. (*Courtesy of* Enrique Pasos, UADY, School of Veterinary Medicine.)

In the bitch, remnant ovarian tissue can develop follicles and corpora lutea, and follicles may become cystic. Because of this, common clinical signs of ROT include periods of vaginal bleeding for several weeks, swelling of the vulva, licking of the vulvar lips, and attraction to males.[3] Occasionally, multifocal areas of erythema are noted on the ventral aspect of the abdomen.[3] Less frequent clinical signs include mammary gland enlargement due to progesterone activity, pollakiuria and stranguria, dermal hyperpigmentation and alopecia, polyuria and polydyspsia, poor coat, weight loss, and recurrent urinary tract infections.[4]

The diagnosis of ROT can be made based on clinical history, clinical symptoms, and routine vaginal cytologic examination (80%–90% superficial cells will indicate an increasing circulating levels of estradiol). When vaginal cytology does not offer satisfactory results or there are still doubts, the levels of 2 ovarian hormones, estradiol and progesterone, can be measured to determine the presence of an ovarian tissue. The use of ultrasonography to diagnose ROT in the dog and cat is limited due to the small size of the remnant tissue. However, it may be useful in medium-sized to large dogs.[5]

The treatment of choice is surgical excision of the remnant tissue. When surgery is not an option or no tissue is found but the problem persists, lifelong therapies are available. Megestrol acetate or mibolerone has been mentioned for use in medical treatment.[6,7] However, several side effects such as mammary gland tumors, acromegaly, clitoral enlargement, and suppression of adrenocortical function may be induced with medical options and caution should be used. The use of a gonadotropin-releasing hormone (GnRH) agonist such as deslorelin is also proposed for medical treatment of ROT but there is not enough medical evidence supporting its efficiency.

In queens, ROT occurs more frequency than in bitches. In this species, revitalization and follicular activity of an ovarian remnant left in the abdominal cavity were shown to occur in the absence of surgical implantation.[8] Clinical signs in the queen can occur several months or years after OVH and include estrus periods with interestrus intervals from 3 weeks to 6 months. Although cats are considered induced

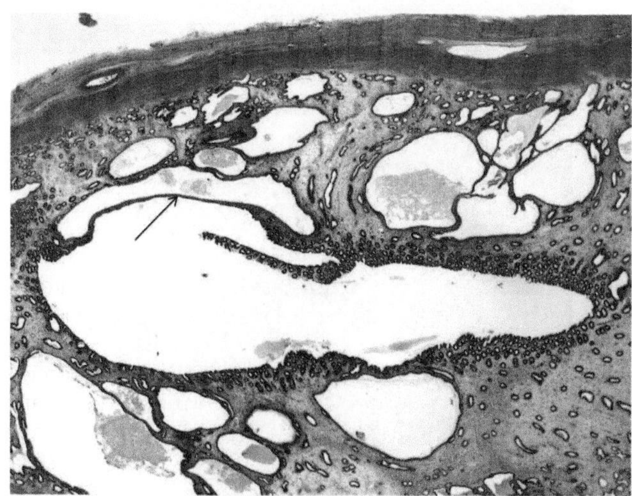

Fig. 3. Photomicrograph of a bitch with cystic endometrial hyperplasia. Endometrial glands are variably dilated and lined by attenuated epithelium (*arrow*). (*Courtesy of* Dr Catherine Lamm, University of Glasgow, School of Veterinary Medicine.)

ovulators, spontaneous ovulations may also occur[9] and prevent queens from entering estrus; cats may show seasonal ovarian activity and seasonal anestrus during late autumn and early winter. Thus, clinical signs of ROT in queens vary year round. Vaginal cytology in a queen with ROT, as in the bitch, reveals many superficial cells indicating estrogenic influence. Stimulation tests using GnRH or human chorionic gonadotropin (hCG) and measuring progesterone concentrations provide a reliable method to diagnose ROT in queens.[10,11] The treatment of choice is surgical. Medical management includes synthetic progestagens,[12] but side effects such as cystic endometrial hyperplasia, pyometra, diabetes, bone marrow toxicity, thyroid dysfunction, and mammary adenoma/fibrosarcoma within others can occur.

Cystic Ovaries

Anovulatory ovarian functional follicular cysts are common incidental findings in older bitches and queens, particularly in those that have never had a litter or may have been single or multiple (**Fig. 1**). Follicular ovarian cysts originate due to failure to ovulate and should be differentiated from other cysts developing from or within the ovaries or the ductal remnants adjacent to them such as cystic rete ovarii, paraovarian cysts, and subsurface epithelial structures (SESs) and from ovarian neoplasias.

In the bitch and queen, clinical signs include persistent or irregular proestrus/estrus manifestations due to hyperestrogenism, anestrus, and infertility. In chronic cases, symmetrical bilateral alopecia and bone marrow suppression may occur; it also predisposes both species to cystic endometrial hyperplasia (CEH)-pyometra complex. In the queen, signs include persistent estrus and aggression even during the

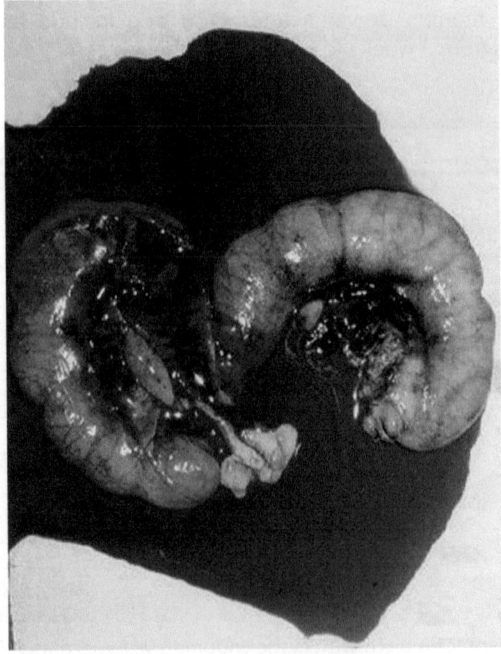

Fig. 4. Recovered uterus of a bitch suffering from pyometra. A bloody to mucopurulent exudate can be appreciated.

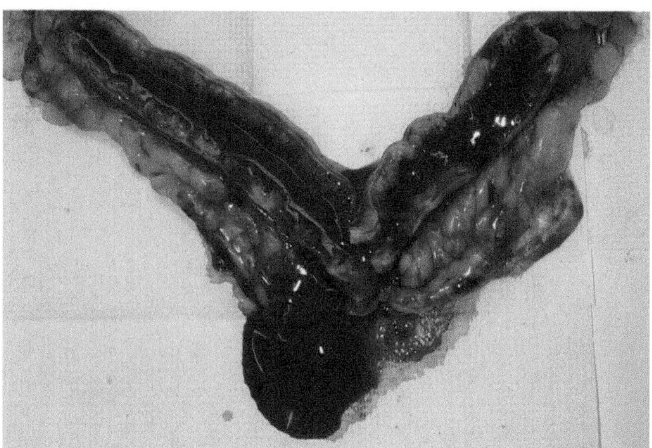

Fig. 5. Recovered uterus of a queen suffering from pyometra. A bloody exudate can be appreciated.

nonseasonal periods of the year; persistent anestrus due to an increase in progesterone secretion does not develop as in bitches since no luteinization of preovulatory follicles occur in this species. The diagnosis is based on vaginal cytology, hormone assays, and ultrasonography. Ovarian ultrasonography will reveal one or more large follicles (1–5 cm in diameter) as hypoechoic to anechoic structures depending on the

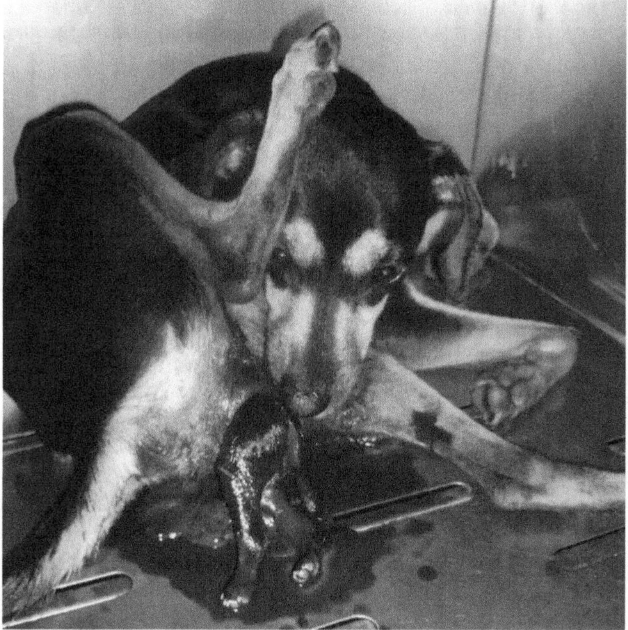

Fig. 6. Dystocia in a bitch predisposing to metritis. Note the thick, dark-brown vaginal discharge and a trapped decomposed pup and placenta.

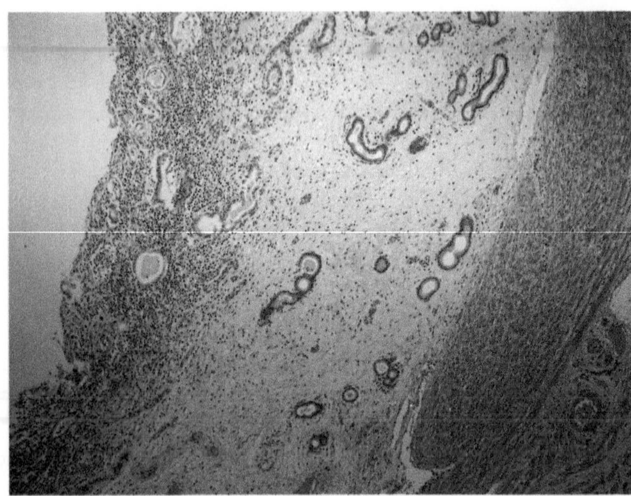

Fig. 7. Photomicrograph of the canine uterus showing a leukocyte infiltration in the endometrium (endometritis). (*Courtesy of* Dr Catherine Lamm, University of Glasgow, School of Veterinary Medicine.)

amount of luteal tissue (**Fig. 2**). Histologic examination of ovarian cysts greatly facilitates distinction between follicular cysts and cysts arising in the rete ovarii, paraovarian cysts, or SESs. However, their functional significance is minimal unless they destroy the adjacent ovarian architecture. Usually, these animals lack clinical signs and ovarian cysts are found incidentally during ultrasound or surgery. The treatment of choice for ovarian follicular cysts is OVH. However, when a single cyst is suspected, laparotomy and cyst rupture may be attempted. Medical treatment includes the induction of ovulation by allowing breeding (in queens) or hormonal therapies with a GnRH and/or hCG.

Differential diagnoses include ovarian tumors, particularly sex-cord stromal tumors such as the granulosa-theca cell tumor, which may be hormone active and produce estrogens. By using medical treatment, the response may allow differentiation of follicular cysts with granulosa-theca cell tumor or other tumors. Other ovarian tumors such as papillary cystadenoma and cystadenocarcinoma occurs commonly in the bitch and may occasionally stimulate the production of ovarian steroids and be involved in CEH.[13]

COMMON LESIONS IN THE UTERUS

Cystic Endometrial Hyperplasia-Pyometra Complex

Pyometra is one of the most common diseases of the uterus in small domestic animals. Literature regarding the cystic endometrial hyperplasia-pyometra complex in dogs and cats is vast and its etiology and pathogenesis have been extensively described.[14–18] The disease is hormone mediated and involves cystic dilatation of endometrial glands; there is accumulation of noninflammatory, watery to viscid, aseptic fluid within the uterine lumen with posterior bacterial contamination, endometrial inflammation, and presence of blood and pus. Pyometra develops in most cases as a consequence of CEH.[17] However, not all cases of CEH will end in pyometra.[14] A second pathologic form of endometrial hyperplasia in the bitch (pseudo-placentational endometrial hyperplasia [PEH]) must be distinguished from

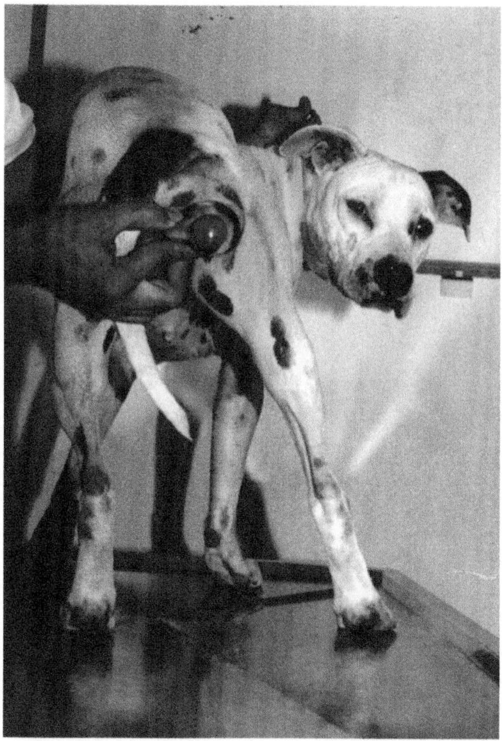

Fig. 8. Vaginal prolapse type I in the bitch.

CEH by the pathologists and clinicians. It also occurs during the luteal phase of the cycle but endometrial proliferation does not involve cystic distention of endometrial glands and is very similar to the normal histology of the endometrium at placentation sites in normal pregnancy.[18] Because of the alteration of the endometrial surface associated with CEH, infertility due to implantation failure after conception can occur[19] (**Fig. 3**). Clinical signs may vary widely depending on the stage of the disease and patency of the cervix; when bacterial replication produce endotoxins, moderate to severe signs of systemic inflammatory response syndrome may be evident.[20] Characteristics of the odorous vaginal discharge may vary from bloody (**Fig. 4**) to bloody mucopurulent depending on whether damage to the endometrial blood vessels has occurred. Ultrasongraphy is the most efficient way to confirm CEH-pyometra cases. The treatment of choice is OVH with prior rehydration and antibiotic therapy. The latest protocols for medical treatment include inhibitors of progesterone receptors such as aglepristone alone[21,22] or in combination with prostaglandin (PG)F2α.[22,23] Aglepristone therapy is also recommended as a preoperative measure to reduce the risk of side effects.

Pyometra is also quite common in the queen, although CEH is not. In the queen, pyometra may occur when cycling at the age of 1 to 10 years or older (mean, 7 years) after a nonfertile breeding. Pathogenicity is similar to that of the bitch but its development is faster (1–4 weeks after estrus) and can also be induced by exogenous administration of progestagens. The frequency of pyometra in queens is lower than that in the bitch because of their special reproductive cycle; queens are seasonal

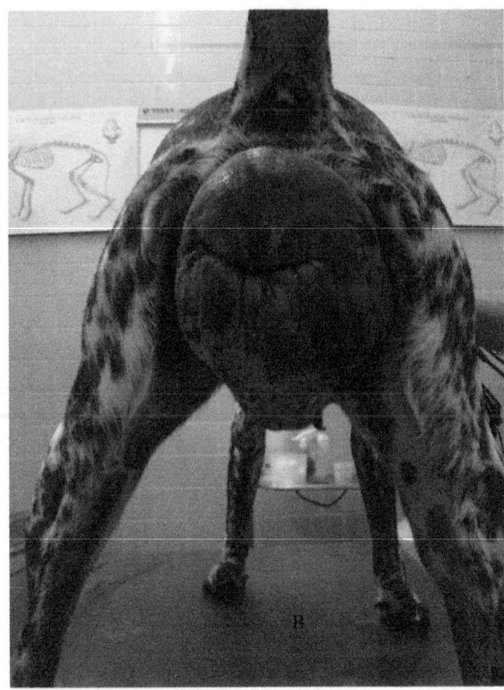

Fig. 9. Vaginal prolapse type III in the bitch.

species and are induced ovulators so there is no prolonged exposure to progesterone as in the dogs. The whole period of progesterone influence over the uterus is shorter (40–50 days) compared to the bitch (over 60 days). Although there is evidence of spontaneous ovulations in queens even in the absence of males,[9,24] the frequency of this event is low. Vaginal discharge may be difficult to detect because of the grooming habits of cats; the discharge is generally purulent and fetid but may vary from bloody to mucoid, to yellow pus or a mixture (**Fig. 5**). Clinical signs associated with pyometra should be differentiated from feline infectious peritonitis. Ultrasound and radiography may indicate a uterine enlargement and may be useful to rule out pregnancy. Treatment of choice is OVH. The progesterone antagonist aglepristone is a new promising approach for the medical treatment of pyometra in this species alone or combined with PGF2α therapy.

Metritis and Endometritis

Metritis is an inflammation of the uterus involving the mucosa and myometrium layers. Unlike pyometra, this is an acute problem generally occurring during the first week postpartum as consequence of bacterial invasion through a dilated cervix to a susceptible uterus. Dogs can have chronic lymphoplasmatic endometritis, not unlike horses, which can result in infertility. It is associated in most cases with dystocia and obstetric manipulation (**Fig. 6**), abortion, retained placenta, or retained dead fetuses. However, in some cases it is produced after natural mating or artificial insemination. In queens, it may also occur in any type of birth. Common isolated bacteria from metritis cases are *Escherichia coli* and *Proteus*, but *Streptococcus* and *Staphylococcus* may also be involved. The infection is limited to the uterus but in unattended

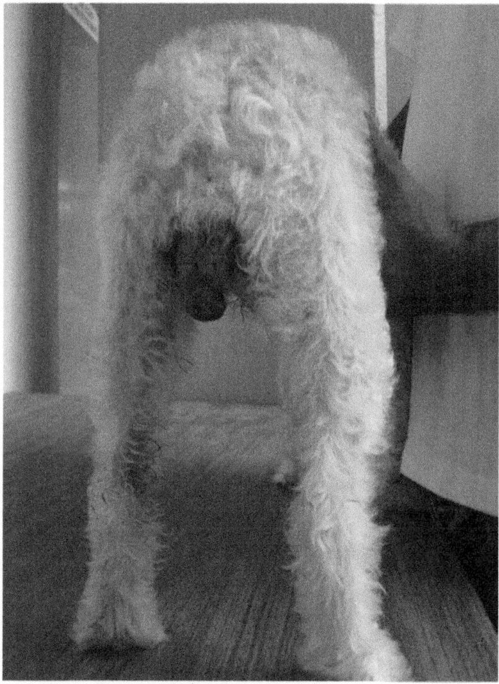

Fig. 10. A case of vulvar canine transmissible venereal tumor in a bitch.

complicated cases can cause a systemic illness leading to septicemia. Acute metritis should be considered in any postpartum animal with signs of systemic illness or with an abnormal vaginal discharge.

Postpartum metritis in the bitch and queen is characterized by a foul-smelling vaginal discharge from purulent to sanguine-purulent. Clinical signs develop very quickly especially when associated with retained fetal membranes; signs include lethargy, anorexia, pyrexia, dehydration, decreased milk production, and abandonment of newborn. Abdominal palpation may reveal a flaccid uterus, and if the presence of a retained fetus or placenta is suspected, an ultrasound and radiology should confirm the diagnosis. Systemic therapies alone or associated with PGF2α have shown consistent positive results. OVH is the last resort when cases become complicated or in animals with refractory cases.

Endometritis (inflammation of the endometrium) is present in many cases of infertile bitches and queens. This is generally chronic and subclinical and must be differentiated from an acute postpartum infection. The histology after recovering the uterus from an OVH (**Fig. 7**) will show an infiltration of polymorphonuclear cells in the endometrium. In the queen with normal ovarian activity, it is associated with infertility and may be more complicated to diagnose than in the bitch, especially when low-grade metritis or a mild infection is present.[25] In the queen, the history of infertility (mating at least 3 times with a fertile male without giving birth) may indicate a uterine infection.[25,26] Therapy using an broad-spectrum antibiotic should be started. Aglepristone together with 15 days of antibiotics has been successfully used in the treatment of endometritis.[27]

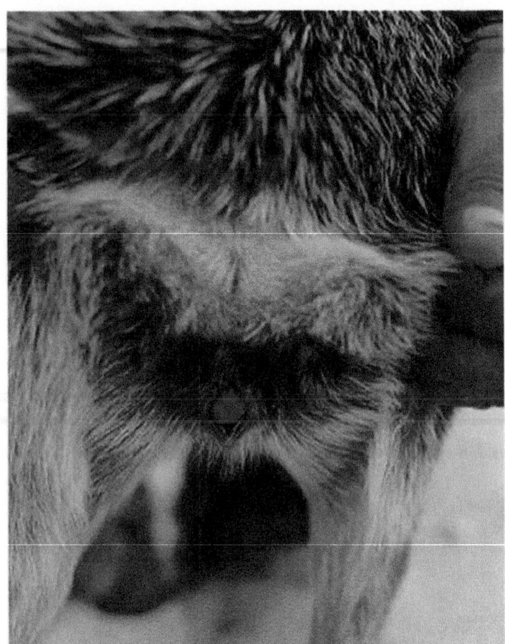

Fig. 11. A case of intersex in a bitch. Note the clitoromegaly.

Uterine Neoplasias and Cysts

Uterine neoplasia occurs infrequently. The majority of uterine tumors in dogs are of mesenchymal origin; they lack a glandular component and are benign. Leiomyomas account for 85% to 90% of all canine uterine tumors and are commonly associated with ovarian follicular cysts, CEH, mammary neoplasia, and hyperplasia.[28] Clinical signs are typically not evident until a uterine tumor reaches a large size. In queens, it may present alterations in the estrus cycle, vaginal discharge, and secondary pyometra.[29] Other less frequent uterine but malignant neoplasms are leiomyosarcoma and carcinoma. Treatment entails OVH.

Endometrial polyps are also seen in old bitches and queens but normally only one develops and they are frequently small and of little consequence unless their growth compromise the uterine lumen.[18] Serosal inclusion cysts may develop in the uterus of the bitch during post partum uterine involution and are incidentally found during OVH or laparotomy.[30] These are frequently submitted as a "lesion of concern," and, except when the structures are of considerable size, they are of minimal clinical significance.

COMMON LESIONS IN THE VAGINA

Vaginal Prolapse

There are several forms of vaginal prolapsed, and the terminology in the literature is often confused. A true vaginal prolapse occurs when the entire vaginal wall extends through the vulvar opening. This condition is rare in the bitch and queen.[31] True vaginal prolapse occurs around parturition, when concentration of serum progesterone declines and the concentration of serum estrogen increase. True vaginal prolapse is graded I through III. Swelling and elevation of the vaginal folds may develop immediately cranial to the urethral orifice (**Fig. 8**) and are categorized as type I. As the

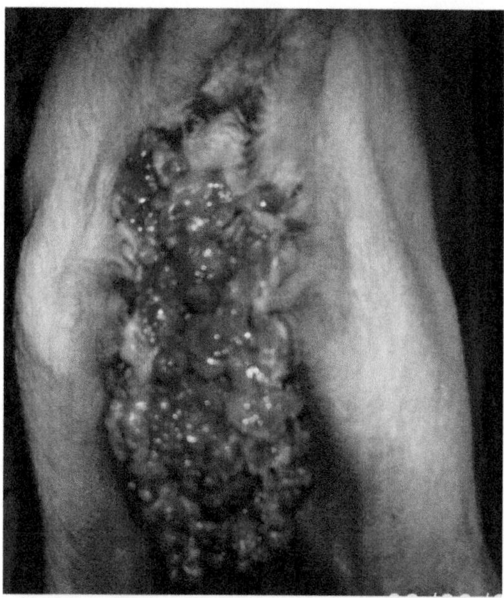

Fig. 12. An extreme case of canine transmissible venereal tumor in the vagina of a dog. (*Courtesy of* Ms Jamie Scott, Private Practice.)

edema progresses, the vagina fold becomes large enough to protrude outside the vulva (type II) until there is a full protrusion of the vaginal circumference through the vulva "donut shaped" (**Fig. 9**) that can cause abrasion of the mucosa and urethral twist (type III). In a type III vaginal prolapse, the urethra may be displaced and twisted and dysuria may occur. The prolapsed vagina is very vulnerable to trauma, ulceration, necrosis, and self-mutilation and may interfere with normal mating. In the queen, vaginal prolapse is very rare and is reported to occur during estrus or anestrus.[32]

Often confused with true vaginal prolapse is the physiologic vaginal protrusion associated with estrogen stimulus during proestrus-estrus. In this case, the tissue is extremely edematous and the vaginal tissue protrudes in thick folds.[33] Vaginal protrusion can be distinguished from a true vaginal prolapse by careful physical examination, clinical history, and knowledge of the stage of cycle.

Vaginal Neoplasia

Vaginal and vulvar neoplasm represents 2.4% to 3% of all tumors in tumor-bearing dogs[34] and the majority of them are benign. Vaginal leiomyomas are among the most common benign tumors in bitches together with fibromas and fibroleiomyomas.[35] Other tumors reported include lipomas, polyps, melanomas, myxomas, and myxofibromas, but these are much less frequent. Canine transmissible venereal tumor (**Fig. 10**) is the most common tumor in the vagina in tropical developing countries,[36] but it is relatively uncommon in the United States and Canada. Clinically, these neoplasms can look similar. Diagnosis is made by physical examination and is confirmed with cytology or histopathology. A prolapsed vagina (see **Fig. 8**) and intersex lesions resulting in clitoromegaly (**Fig. 11**) can be mistaken with tumors. Most vaginal neoplasms behave in a benign fashion and complete surgical resection is usually curative. In the case of transmissible venereal tumor when tumors are too large (**Fig. 12**), chemotherapy is compulsory. In queens, vaginal tumors are uncommon and may be found in healthy animals; benign leiomyomas are the most commonly reported.[37,38]

SUMMARY

Lesions on the reproductive tract are common findings in small animal practice. Some of these lesions, such as pyometra and metritis, can seriously affect the reproductive capacity of the bitch and queen and, if not recognized and treated early, can lead to mortality. Clinicians must be aware of the different reproductive lesions and be prepared to differentiate those of concern and identify which require treatment.

REFERENCES

1. Wallace MS. The ovarian remnant syndrome in the bitch and queen. Vet Clin North Am 1991;21:501–7.
2. Terazono T, Inoue M, Kaedei Y, et al. Assessment of canine ovaries autografted to various body sites. Theriogenology 2012;77:131–8.
3. Sangster C. Ovarian remnant syndrome in a 5-year-old bitch. Can Vet J 2005;46: 62–4.
4. Ball RL, Birchard SJ, May LR, et al. Ovarian remnant syndrome in dogs and cats: 21 cases (2000–2007). J Am Vet Med Assoc 2010;236:548–53.
5. Sontas BH, Gürbulak K, Ekici H. Síndrome de remanente ovárico en la perra: revisión bibliográfica. Arch Med Vet 2007;39:99–104.
6. Romagnoli S. Ovarian remnant syndrome. Proceedings of fourth EVSSAR Congress, Barcelona (Spain), 2004. p. 239–41.
7. Johnston SD, Kustritz MVR, Olson PNS. Ovarian remnant syndrome. In: Johnston SD, Root Kustritz MV, Olson PNS, editors. Canine and feline theriogenology. Philadelphia: WB Saunders; 2001. p. 199–200.
8. De Nardo GA, Becker K, Brown NO, et al. Ovarian remnant syndrome: revascularization of free-floating ovarian tissue in the feline abdominal cavity. J Am Anim Hosp Assoc 2001;37:290–6.
9. Concannon PW, Verstegen J. Some unique aspects of canine and feline female reproduction important in veterinary practice. In: Proceedings of the 30th World Small Animal Veterinary Congress. Mexico City (Mexico): 2005.
10. England GCW. Confirmation of ovarian remnant syndrome in the queen using hCG administration. Vet Rec 1997;141:309–10.
11. Scebra LR, Griffin B. Evaluation of a commercially available luteinizing hormone test to distinguish between ovariectomized and sexually intact queens. In: Proceedings of the 21st Annual Meeting of the American College of Veterinary Internal Medicine Forum. Charlotte (NC): 2003. p. 4–7.
12. Burke TJ, Reynolds HA, Sokolowski JH. A 280-day tolerance-efficacy study with mibolerone for suppression of estrus in the cat. Am J Vet Res 1977;38:469–77.
13. Schlafer DH, Miller RB. Female genital system. In: Maxie MG, editor. Jubb, Kennedy and Palmer's pathology of domestic animals, vol. 3. Edinburgh: Saunders-Elsevier; 2007. p. 429–564.
14. De Bosschere H, Ducatelle R, Vermeirsch H, et al. Cystic endometrial hyperplasia-pyometra complex in the bitch: should the two entities be disconnected? Theriogenology 2001;55:1509–19.
15. Arora N, Sandford J, Browning GF, et al. A model for cystic endometrial hyperplasia/pyometra complex in the bitch. Theriogenology 2006;66:1530–6.
16. Smith FO. Canine pyometra. Theriogenology 2006;66:610–2.

17. Pretzer SD. Clinical presentation of canine pyometra and mucometra: a review. Theriogenology 2008;70, 359–63.
18. Schlafer DH, Gifford AT. Cystic endometrial hyperplasia, pseudo-placentational endometrial hyperplasia, and other cystic conditions of the canine and feline uterus Theriogenology 2008;70:349–58.
19. Freshman JL. Clinical approach to infertility in the cycling bitch. Vet Clin North Am 1991;21:427–35.
20. Purvis D, Kirby R. Systemic inflammatory response syndrome: Septic shock. Vet Clin North Am Small Anim Pract 1994;24:1225–47.
21. Trasch K, Wehrend A, Bostedt H. Follow-up examinations of bitches after conservative treatment of pyometra with the antigestagen aglepristone. J Vet Med Assoc 2003;50:375–9.
22. Fieni F. Clinical evaluation of the use of aglepristone, with or without cloprostenol, to treat cystic endometrial hyperplasia-pyometra complex in bitches. Theriogenology 2006;66:1550–6.
23. Gobello C, Castex G, Klima L, et al. A study of two protocols combining aglepristone and cloprostenol to treat open cervix pyometra in the bitch. Theriogenology 2003;60: 901–8.
24. Lowler DF, Johnston SD, Hegstad RL, et al. Ovulation without cervical stimulation in domestic cats. J Rep Fertil Suppl 1993;47:57–61.
25. Axner E, Agren E, Baverud V, et al. Infertility in the cycling queen: seven cases. J Feline Med Surg 2008;10:566–76.
26. Axner E. Updates of reproductive physiology, genital diseases and artificial insemination in the domestic cat. Reprod Dom Anim 2008;43(Suppl 2):144–9.
27. Fontaine E, Levy X, Grellet A, et al. Diagnosis of endometritis in the bitch: A new approach. Reprod Dom Anim 2009;44(Suppl 2):196–9.
28. Klein MK. Tumors of the female reproductive system. In: Withrow SJ, MacEwen EG, editors. Small animal clinical oncology. 3rd edition. Philadelphia: Saunders; 2001. p. 445–54.
29. Stein BS. Tumors of the feline genital tract. J Am Anim Hosp Assoc 1981;17:1022–5.
30. Johnston SD, Root-Kustritz MV, Olson PNS. Disorders of canine uterus and uterine tubes (oviducts). In: Canine and feline theriogenology. Philadelphia: WB Saunders; 2001. p. 206–24.
31. Alan M, Cetin Y, Sendag S, et al. True vaginal prolapsed in a bitch. Anim Reprod Sci 2007;100:411–4.
32. Johnston SD, Root Kustritz MV, Olson PNS. Disorders of the feline vagina, vestibule, and vulva. In: Canine and feline theriogenology. Philadelphia: WB Saunders; 2001. p. 472–3.
33. Purswell BJ. Vaginal disorders. In: Ettinger SJ, Feldman EC, editors. Textbook of veterinary internal medicine. Philadelphia: WB Saunders; 2000. p. 1566–71.
34. McEntee M. Reproductive oncology. Clin Tech Small Anim Pract 2002;17:133–49.
35. Thacher C, Bradley RL. Vulvar and vaginal tumors in the dog: a retrospective study. J Am Vet Med Assoc 1983;183:690–2.
36. Ortega-Pacheco A, Segura-Correa J, Jimenez-Coello M, et al. Reproductive patterns and reproductive pathologies of stray bitches in the tropics. Theriogenology 2002;67: 382–90.
37. Wolke RE. Vaginal leiomyoma as a cause of chronic constipation in a cat. J Am Vet Med Assoc 1963;143:1103–5.
38. Whitehead JE. Neoplasia in the cat. Vet Med Small Anim Clin 1967;62:357.

Bacterial Reproductive Pathogens of Cats and Dogs

Elizabeth M. Graham, MVB, MVM, PhD, MRCVS[a,*],
David J. Taylor, MA, PhD, VetMB, MRCVS[b]

KEYWORDS

• Feline • Canine • Infectious disease • Theriogenology
• Bacteria • Urogenital flora

With the notable exception of *Brucella canis* in dogs, exogenous bacterial pathogens are sporadic causes of reproductive disease in cats and dogs. Most commonly, bacterial infection of the reproductive tract is endogenous in origin; many of the bacteria etiologically involved in reproductive disease form part of the urogenital microflora (**Table 1**). Bacterial reproductive disease is therefore frequently opportunistic, and predisposing factors must be present for disease to develop (**Table 2**).

Culture, polymerase chain reaction (PCR), and serology are commonly used to diagnose bacterial reproductive disease, but the limitations of each method must be understood. The presence of a urogenital microflora must be considered when interpreting culture results from vaginal and seminal secretions; furthermore, age, antimicrobial treatment, and stage of the estrus cycle will influence the quantity and quality of bacterial isolates.[1–4] Isolation of pure profuse cultures, absence of other pathogens, supportive cytological assessment, and response to antimicrobial treatment may all be helpful in establishing a causal role for any recovered organisms.[5] Isolation of bacteria from sites that are normally sterile, such as blood or parenchymatous organs, together with supportive histopathology, provides a definitive diagnosis. For exogenous infections, PCR presents a rapid and sensitive alternative to culture. However, false-positive results can arise from laboratory contamination, particularly with "open tube" techniques. Serologic evidence of exposure can be useful in diagnosing exogenous infection; assay specificity and timing of sampling are critical.

The authors have nothing to disclose.
[a] School of Veterinary Medicine, College of Medical, Veterinary and Life Sciences, University of Glasgow, Bearsden Road, Glasgow G61 1QH, UK
[b] 31 North Birbiston Road, Lennoxtown, Glasgow G66 7LZ, UK
* Corresponding author.
E-mail address: libby.graham@glasgow.ac.uk

Vet Clin Small Anim 42 (2012) 561–582
doi:10.1016/j.cvsm.2012.01.013
vetsmall.theclinics.com
0195-5616/12/$ – see front matter

Table 1
Bacteria isolated from the prepuce and vagina of clinically healthy dogs and cats

Prepuce		Vagina	
Male Dog[37]	**Tom**[37,103]	**Bitch**[3,37,104,105]	**Queen**[1,37,103]
Staphylococcus spp Coagulase-neg. staphylococci Coagulase-pos. staphylococci	*Staphylococcus* spp Coagulase-neg. staphylococci	*Staphylococcus* spp Coagulase-neg. staphylococci Coagulase-pos. staphylococci	*Staphylococcus* spp Coagulase-neg. staphylococci Coagulase-pos. staphylococci
Streptococcus spp β-hemolytic streptococci α-hemolytic streptococci Nonhemolytic streptococci	*Streptococcus* spp β-hemolytic streptococci α-hemolytic streptococci Nonhemolytic streptococci	*Streptococcus* spp β-hemolytic streptococci α-hemolytic streptococci Nonhemolytic streptococci	*Streptococcus* spp β-hemolytic streptococci α-hemolytic streptococci Nonhemolytic streptococci
Corynebacterium spp	*Corynebacterium* spp	*Corynebacterium* spp	*Corynebacterium* spp
Escherichia coli	*Escherichia coli*	*Escherichia coli*	*Escherichia coli*
Pasteurella spp	*Pasteurella* spp	*Pasteurella* spp	*Pasteurella* spp
Mycoplasma spp	*Mycoplasma* spp	*Mycoplasma* spp	*Mycoplasma* spp
Haemophilus spp	*Moraxella/Brahamella* spp	*Haemophilus* spp	*Haemophilus* spp
Klebsiella pneumoniae	*Bacteroides* spp	*Klebsiella* spp	*Klebsiella* spp
Acinetobacter spp	*Fusobacterium* spp	*Acinetobacter* spp	*Acinetobacter* spp
Moraxella spp	*Simonsiella* spp	*Moraxella* spp	*Bacteroides* spp
Proteus spp		*Bacteroides* spp	*Peptococcus* spp

Bacillus spp	*Fusobacterium* spp	*Arcanobacterium pyogenes*
Pseudomonas spp	*Peptostreptococcus* spp	*Lactobacillus* spp
Enterococcus spp	*Proteus* spp	
Ureaplasma spp	*Bacillus* spp	
Flavobacterium spp	*Pseudomonas* spp	
	Enterococcus spp	
	Ureaplasma spp	
	Flavobacterium spp	
	Citrobacter spp	
	Clostridium spp	
	Neisseria spp	
	Enterobacter spp	
	Micrococcus spp	
	Alcaligenes faecalis	
	Prevotella spp	

Adapted from Barsanti JA. Genitourinary infections. In: Greene CE, editor. Infectious diseases of the dog and cat. 3rd edition. Philadelphia: Saunders Elsevier; 1996. p. 935–61; with permission.

Table 2
Predisposing factors for infection with endogenous reproductive bacterial pathogens

Clinical Disease	Predisposing Factors[37,45,106]
Vaginitis	• Congenital anatomic abnormalities (eg, stenosis) • Vaginal atrophy following ovariohysterectomy • Immaturity • Neoplasia • Trauma • Foreign body • Drugs • UTI • Pyometra • Systemic disease (eg, diabetes) • Primary viral infection
Metritis	• Trauma (eg, dystocia, obstetric manipulation) • Abortion • Retention of fetal or placental tissue
Pyometra	• Middle-aged intact bitch • Unbred intact queen >3-yr-old • Unsuccessful matings (queen) • Exogenous progestins
Mastitis	• Trauma to teat and overlying skin • Poor hygiene • Retention of secretions
Epididymitis-Orchitis	• Trauma • Concurrent cystitis or prostatitis
Prostatitis	• Intact male • Concurrent cystitis or pyelonephritis • Disease of prostatic urethra (eg, urethral urolithiasis) • Disease that interferes with prostatic fluid formation and secretion (eg, prostatic neoplasia)
Neonatal disease	• Dystocia • Hypothermia • Poor hygiene • Overcrowding • Insufficient passive immunity • Low body weight • Prematurity • Juvenile queen where GGS endemic • Immature immune system • Mastitis or metritis in dam • Antimicrobial treatment suppressing colonization resistance

BRUCELLA CANIS

Brucella spp are small, aerobic gram-negative coccobacilli, which stain red using the modified Ziehl-Neelsen (MZN) technique. In addition to *B canis,* dogs can be infected with *B abortus, B melitensis,* and *B suis.*[6–8] *Brucella* is not an important cause of reproductive disease in the cat.[9] However, productive infections can occur; a cat infected with *B suis* was identified as the source of an outbreak of brucellosis in 6 human contacts.[10]

Seroprevalence studies indicate that canine brucellosis is widespread in the southern US, Central and Southern America, and Asia.[11] Sporadic cases have been reported in Europe. *Brucella* is under statutory control in the UK; the only confirmed case of *B canis* infection was diagnosed post quarantine in a dog imported from Spain.[12] *Brucella* has a predilection for male and female reproductive tracts in sexually mature animals. Infection is acquired by inhalation, ingestion, and insemination; significantly, infection can also be transmitted in utero. Invading bacteria survive phagocytosis[13] and are transported to the uterus, epididymides, and prostate via a cell-associated bacteremia 2 weeks post infection (PI). Bacteremia persists for at least 6 months PI and can be detected for up to 64 months.[14]

Vaginal and seminal secretions from infected animals contain the highest bacterial loads and are therefore the most significant sources of infection.[14] Bacteriuria persists for at least 3 months PI, facilitating horizontal transmission between male dogs. Although bacteria are shed in feces, milk, saliva, and nasal and ocular secretions, these are not regarded as major sources of infection. Infection can also be acquired indirectly; *B abortus* can survive in water and damp soil for up to 4 months, and *B canis* remains viable in semen and mouse cryoprotective agent for up to 48 hours.[15,16]

Clinical Signs

The clinical signs associated with *Brucella* infection are not pathognomonic. Infected animals are rarely systemically ill and fever is very uncommon, perhaps because this organism lacks the lipopolysaccharide (LPS) antigen associated with endotoxemia.[17] Clinical signs can also reflect localization of the bacteria in extrareproductive tract sites such as the eye, intervertebral disc spaces, and reticuloendothelial system.[18,19]

Brucellosis causes spontaneous late abortion in an otherwise healthy bitch. This most commonly occurs from days 30 to 57, peaking between days 45 and 55.[20] Abortion is usually accompanied by a vaginal discharge lasting up to 6 weeks. Earlier abortions can occur but may be incorrectly reported as conception failure since the bitch typically ingests aborted fetuses. Early embryonic death and fetal resorption can occur 10 to 20 days post-mating. Many bitches that abort will subsequently have normal litters, although some may experience intermittent reproductive failures.[21] Some litters born to infected bitches contain both live and dead pups, although most live pups die shortly thereafter. Those that survive suffer generalized lymphadenopathy and persistent hyperglobulinemia, and they develop clinical disease on reaching sexual maturity.[14]

Clinical signs of epididymitis become apparent from week 5 PI. In acute infection, scrotal distention caused by enlargement of the tail of the epididymis and accumulation of serosanguineous fluid is clinically evident. Primary orchitis is not common but can occur.[22,23] Infected dogs may also present with scrotal dermatitis caused by constant licking of the scrotal skin and secondary bacterial infection.[21] Unilateral or bilateral testicular atrophy develops in chronic infection. Sperm abnormalities are detectable with the onset of clinical signs, with over 90% abnormal by week 20. Concurrent prostatitis is also common.[22]

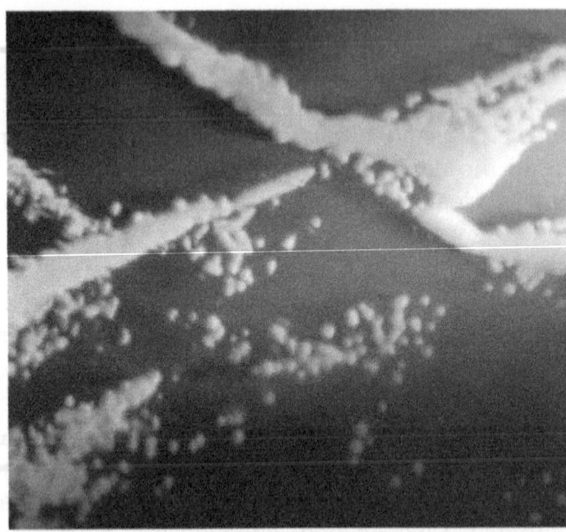

Fig. 1. A 48-hour culture of *B canis* on serum dextrose agar (SDA) incubated in air under 10% CO_2 at 37°C. *B canis* is slow-growing and the characteristic "rough" colonies do not appear before 48 hours on solid media. (*Image courtesy of* Lorraine Perrett, Animal Health and Veterinary Laboratories Agency [AHVLA], Weybridge, Surrey, UK.)

Diagnosis

Isolation and identification of *B canis* is the gold standard (**Fig. 1**). Placenta, lymph nodes, prostate, and spleen are suitable samples for culture, whereas semen, vaginal secretions, and urine (unless collected by cystocentesis) are frequently contaminated with other organisms. Blood submitted in an aerobic blood culture bottle is the sample of choice because of the lack of contaminating organisms and prolonged bacteremia. Culture is time-consuming and presents a potential biohazard to laboratory personnel, necessitating Containment Level 3 (CL3) facilities (**Table 3**).

PCR can be a rapid, highly sensitive and specific assay and presents a useful alternative to culture for the direct detection of *Brucella*. Most PCR assays are designed to detect gene sequences conserved across all *Brucella* species and biovars, and therefore detect *Brucella* to genus level only. A multiplex PCR assay that can differentiate all known species, including *B canis,* has recently been published.[24] In dogs, *Brucella* DNA has been detected in whole blood, serum, semen, vaginal swabs, inguinal lymph nodes, and aqueous humor.[16,18,25–27] Compared to blood culture, the diagnostic sensitivity of whole blood PCR was 100% in naturally infected dogs.[25] However, some dogs were PCR positive and blood culture negative, which likely reflects the lower sensitivity of blood culture.[28]

Serology is widely used to diagnose canine brucellosis. An understanding of assay sensitivity and specificity, the chronology of antibody development, and the antigen used are all required to successfully interpret test results. Antibodies are not detectable for 3 to 4 weeks PI, and occasionally up to 12 weeks PI.[14] False-positive reactions can be problematic since epitopes within the LPS antigens are frequently shared with other bacterial species. The most commonly used antigens are *B ovis* or *B canis* LPS antigens; assays based on the *B canis* nonpathogenic (M–) strains are more specific.[29]

The rapid slide agglutination test (RSAT) is a simple, rapid, and sensitive test designed to detect antibodies to *Brucella* LPS antigen. This is most accurate as a screening test from 8 to 12 weeks PI. The 2ME-RSAT is considered more specific

Table 3
Diagnosis of major bacterial reproductive pathogens by culture

Pathogen	Optimal Samples	Direct Microscopy	Culture Time	Additional Tests	Comments	Alternative Tests
Brucella	• Blood • Placenta	• MZN-positive clusters of cells	• Min. 48 hr	• Multiplex PCR • Serotyping	• Exogenous • CL3 Laboratory • Selective media • Reportable in UK	• AGID (serum) • PCR (whole blood, tissues, secretions)
Escherichia coli	• Genital swabs • Neonatal tissues • Milk	• Gram-negative rods	• Min. 24–48 hr	• API 20E	• Endogenous	• N/A
Streptococcus	• Genital swabs • Placenta • Fetal tissues • Neonatal tissues	• Gram-positive cocci in chains or pairs	• Min. 24–48 hr	• API 20 Strep • Lancefield Grouping	• Endogenous	• N/A
Leptospira	• Urine • Fetal tissues	• Motile helical bacteria using dark ground microscopy	• Min. 2–6 wk	• Serotyping • DNA profiling	• Exogenous • CL3 Laboratory • Selective media • Fragile	• MAT (serum) • PCR (tissues, urine) • FA (tissues)
Salmonella	• Placenta • Fetal tissues • Genital swabs	• Gram-negative rods	• Min. 48 hr	• API 20E • Serotyping • Phage typing	• Exogenous • Selective media	• PCR (feces, tissues)
Campylobacter	• Placenta • Fetal tissues • Genital swabs	• Slender, curved Gram-negative rods	• Min. 48 hr	• API Campy	• Exogenous • Selective media • Microaerobic	• PCR (feces, tissues)
Staphylococcus	• Genital swabs • Neonatal tissues • Milk	• Gram-positive cocci in bunches of grapes	• Min. 24–48 hr	• ID32*Staphylococcus* • DNAse test • Coagulase test	• Endogenous	• N/A

than the RSAT, as 2-mercaptoethanol (2-ME) destroys cross-reacting IgM antibodies. Agar gel immunodiffusion (AGID) detects precipitating antibodies against *Brucella* cell wall or cytoplasmic antigen. The assay is highly specific for *Brucella* spp, particularly if based on the *B canis* cytoplasmic antigens (CPag). CPag antibodies are detectable from 8 to 12 weeks PI and can persist for up to 36 months after bacteremia has resolved, making the test useful for detecting chronic infections.[14] The AGID assay is frequently used as a confirmatory test for other serologic assays.[30] Enzyme-linked immunosorbent assays (ELISAs) have been developed to detect antibodies to *B canis* cell wall, cytoplasmic, and recombinant antigens and may prove a simpler and more rapid alternative to agglutination assays. A recently described ELISA based on heat-soluble *B canis* antigen was highly sensitive (91.1%) and specific (100%) compared to AGID.[30] Samples with positive or equivocal results on serology should be submitted for a direct confirmatory method given the propensity for inaccurate results. Preliminary PCR data suggest that the 2ME-RSAT and AGID may be less sensitive but more specific than previously reported.[31]

Antimicrobial Therapy and Control

Brucellosis is problematic to treat, given the inability of many antimicrobials to attain adequate concentrations at intracellular level. No antimicrobial protocol has been shown to consistently achieve a long-term cure. Combination therapy is frequently recommended; the most efficacious is reported to be a combination of tetracyclines and aminoglycosides, or fluoroquinolones and aminoglycosides.[11,18,32] Where *Brucella* is identified within kennels, a test and elimination strategy can be instigated. To prevent new infections, all incoming animals should be isolated until 2 seronegative tests are returned 30 days apart.[14] Prebreeding tests should also be carried out.[11]

B canis is not considered a significant zoonosis under normal circumstances, with infections reported to be mild and uncommon. However, serious illness can occur in immunocompromised patients.[33] Infection is usually transmitted by direct contact with infected animals or through occupational aerosol exposure. The true incidence of infection is unknown as clinical signs are usually nonspecific, and diagnosis is challenging.

ESCHERICHIA COLI

Escherichia coli is a facultatively anaerobic, gram-negative member of the Enterobacteriaceae family. *E coli* forms part of the intestinal microflora in all mammals and can also be isolated from healthy epithelial tissues. *E coli* is one of the most frequently isolated bacteria from the lower urogenital tract in clinically healthy cats and dogs.

E coli infections of the reproductive tract are opportunistic infections caused by strains within the gastrointestinal (GI) microflora. In humans, 2 distinct groups of *E coli* reside in the healthy GI tract: commensal strains that rarely cause disease and pathogenic strains with potential to cause disease at any site external to the GI tract. The latter are called extraintestinal pathogenic *E coli* (ExPEC). These strains possess a toolkit of virulence genes that encode resistance to host defenses (eg, capsular K antigen), iron-acquisition systems (eg, aerobactin), adhesins (eg, P fimbriae), and exotoxins (eg, hemolysins).[34] It is likely that equivalent groups of *E coli* reside in the canine and feline GI tracts and that many *E coli* infections of the reproductive tract are caused by ExPEC strains. It is known that *E coli* isolates recovered from bitches with pyometra are derived from the GI microflora[35] and carry a wide range of virulence genes, including uropathogenic specific protein (*usp*), cytotoxin necrotizing factor (*cnf-1*), β-hemolysin (*hlyA*), and P fimbriae (*papC*) genes.[36] Additional research is required to ascertain whether a particular combination of virulence genes can accurately define ExPEC strains.

While only virulent *E coli* isolates secrete exotoxins, all *E coli* strains release endotoxin on cell lysis. Endotoxin can activate the host systemic inflammatory response syndrome (SIRS) on entering the systemic circulation. Uncontrolled SIRS can trigger sepsis and multiorgan failure, and endotoxemia is a potentially fatal sequel to pyometra, metritis, neonatal bacteremia, and mastitis caused by *E coli*.

Clinical Signs

E coli is a common cause of vaginitis, metritis, mastitis, and pyometra in bitches and queens and is an uncommon cause of abortion.[37] A wide range of vaginal microflora organisms have been recovered from pyometra cases, with *E coli* isolated from 70%.[2,38,39] Peak binding of *E coli* to the endometrium occurs in the early luteal phase,[40] when bitches are most vulnerable to the development of pyometra.[41] *E coli* can be isolated from the healthy uterus during proestrus and estrus,[1,3] which may provide a residual source of infection. Concurrent urinary tract infection (UTI) with identical strains of *E coli* is common,[35,40,42] but it is unclear whether UTI predisposes to, or is a consequence of, pyometra. Endotoxin is abortifacient in other species and has been cited as a possible cause of partial abortion in a bitch.[43] However, *E coli* does not appear to be a common cause of abortion in cats and dogs.[44]

Most cases of epididymitis, orchitis, and prostatitis in companion animals are bacterial in origin, with *E coli* most frequently isolated.[37] Infection can affect 1 or all 3 organs. In most cases, infection ascends from the distal urethra with concurrent UTI commonly reported. None of these conditions are common in companion animals, particularly the cat.

Disease and death are common in neonatal pups or kittens (days 0–14). Infectious diseases of bacterial origin are the second most common cause of death after dystocia, with *E coli* and β-hemolytic (βH) *Streptococcus* spp the most significant bacterial pathogens. Puppies and kittens are colonized with *E coli* in their first 24 hours, most commonly from maternal vaginal discharges and from the environment; over 60% of *E coli* strains isolated from pups were identical to strains isolated from dams and other dogs in the kennel.[45] Under normal circumstances, colonization should be asymptomatic or cause mild self-limiting disease. However, the presence of predisposing factors can trigger bacteremia and endotoxemia (**Table 2**). It is not yet clear whether particular virulent strains of *E coli* are consistently involved.

Diagnosis

E coli is readily cultured from clinical specimens using routine diagnostic media (**Fig. 2**). PCR can be used to detect virulence genes present in *E coli* isolates,[36] but additional research is needed to identify the combination of genes that define virulent strains before such assays can provide useful information to veterinary practitioners.

Antimicrobial Treatment and Control

Sensitivity testing should be carried out if antimicrobial therapy is indicated, as antimicrobial resistant isolates are increasingly prevalent.[46] A recent study monitoring *E coli* isolates from healthy dogs in the United Kingdom (N = 183), found that 29% of healthy dogs were shedding isolates resistant to at least one antimicrobial, with 15% carrying multidrug-resistant (MDR) isolates. Resistance to ampicillin, tetracycline, and trimethoprim was most prevalent.[47] To control disease, predisposing causes must be identified and minimized.

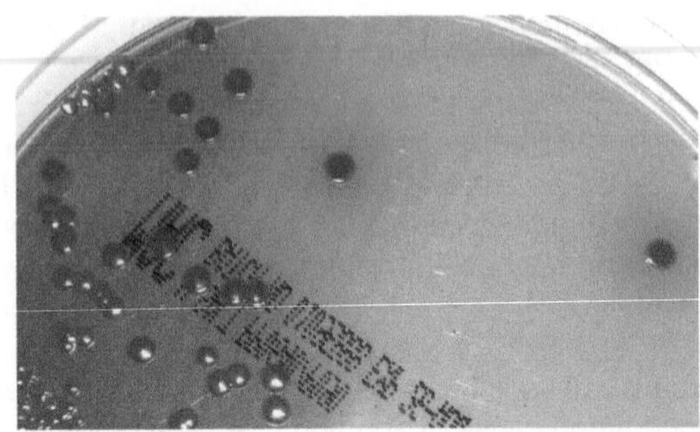

Fig. 2. *E coli* is a strong lactose fermenter, producing bright pink colonies on MacConkey agar within 24 hours. Identification based on biochemical properties can be made using the Analytical Profile Index (API) numerical system (API 20E; bioMérieux, Marcy l'Etoile, France).

Animal handlers and veterinarians are potentially at risk from ExPEC strains. Virulence factors detected in strains carried by healthy dogs are known to be significant in human infections.[36] Furthermore, MDR organisms and resistance plasmids could readily be transferred between species and organisms, respectively. MDR ExPEC strains (ST131) have been detected in both clinical and healthy companion animal samples.[48]

STREPTOCOCCUS

Streptococcus spp are small, nonmotile, facultatively anaerobic gram-positive cocci, which frequently appear in chains in clinical specimens (**Fig. 3**). Many species form part of the canine and feline microflora populating skin and mucous membranes.

Streptococci are common opportunistic pathogens in animals and humans, and predisposing factors for infection are listed in **Table 2**. Streptococci can be categorized in several ways—first, by their effect on erythrocytes in culture medium; most pathogenic streptococci are βH, whereas α-hemolytic and non-hemolytic organisms are less likely to be clinically significant. Streptococcal species are also categorized by antigenic differences in their cell wall C-substance (Lancefield groups). In both cats and dogs, clinical

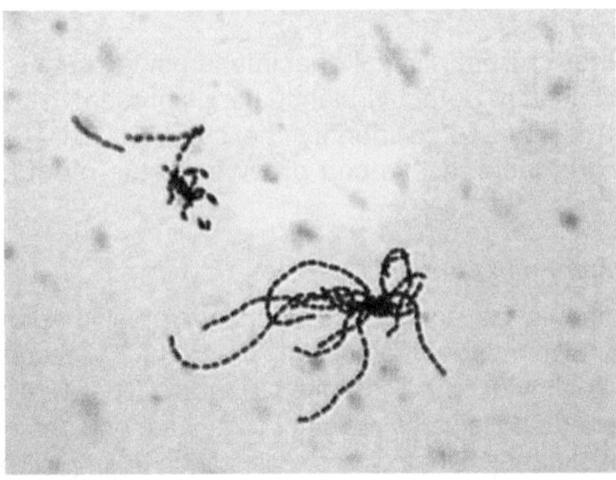

Fig. 3. *S canis* manifests as gram-positive cocci in chains or pairs in smears made from clinical specimens or isolates.

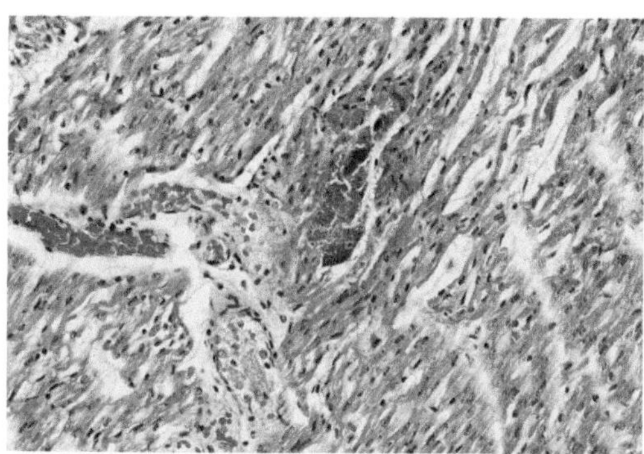

Fig. 4. Gram-positive cocci within cardiac tissue from a case of neonatal septicemia. *βH Streptococcus* sp was subsequently isolated from this sample. (*Image courtesy of* Dr Catherine Lamm, University of Glasgow.)

disease is most commonly associated with Lancefield group G streptococci (GGS), predominantly *S canis*. However, some organisms within Lancefield groups B (GBS), C (GCS), L (GLS), and M (GMS) have been etiologically associated with neonatal septicemia, abortion, and endometritis.[49–53]

Clinical Signs

In the past, βH streptococci have been linked to multiple diseases of the reproductive tract, including infertility. However, many early reports need to be interpreted carefully, given the frequency with which βH streptococci can be isolated from the urogenital tracts of clinically healthy animals. Currently, there is little causal evidence to link βH streptococci with infertility in the bitch or the queen.[54] Nonetheless, βH streptococci are a recognized cause of metritis, pyometra, placentitis, and abortion,[38,50,52,54] usually as a result of ascending infection. βH streptococci have also been isolated from sporadic cases of mastitis and vaginitis.[55,56]

βH streptococci are a major cause of neonatal death. Typically, neonates become infected from the maternal birth canal via the umbilicus or, less commonly, from mastitic milk.[57,58] GGS bacteria predominate, with *S canis* the most frequently identified species.[53] However, many isolates are identified only to genus level. *S canis* septicemia is a particularly well-described problem in breeding catteries.[54] Several kittens in a litter can be infected at once, most commonly the first litter of a young queen. Young queens have higher bacterial loads in the vagina, which persist throughout pregnancy, whereas older queens can eliminate infection by mid-gestation.

βH streptococci were causally associated with all 24 canine fetal or neonatal deaths investigated over a 33-month period in a regional diagnostic laboratory.[59] Many isolates were not speciated; of those that were, *S canis* predominated (**Fig. 4**). GBS and GCS are rare causes of reproductive disease in cats and dogs. *S agalactiae* (GBS) caused neonatal septicemia in 2 litters of pups in a research colony. One bitch presented systemically ill with a purulent vaginal discharge; the other bitch remained well. The organism was isolated from vaginal swabs and pup tissues.[51] *S dysgalactiae* subsp *dysgalactiae* (GCS) was isolated in pure culture from neonatal puppies that died of septicemia within 72 hours of birth.[49]

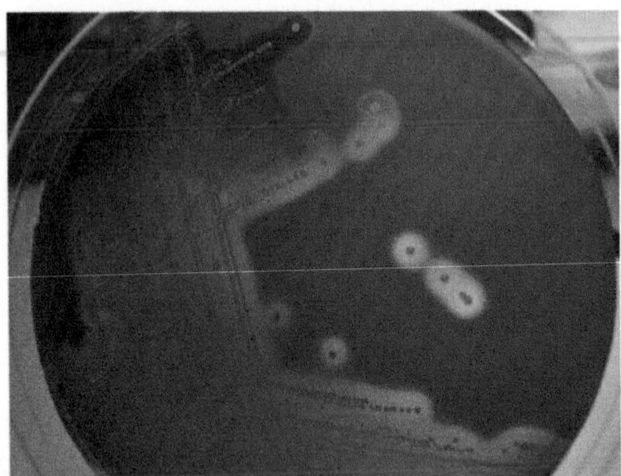

Fig. 5. *S canis* is βH on sheep blood agar, producing a wide zone of clear hemolysis. Lancefield group testing can be carried out on isolates using commercial agglutination kits or the ring precipitation test. Principal species can be distinguished biochemically using the API 20S numerical system.

Diagnosis

Samples should be submitted in transport medium as streptococci are susceptible to desiccation.[60] Streptococci are readily cultured from clinical specimens using routine diagnostic media. βH species produce a clear zone of hemolysis on blood agar within 24 to 48 hours (**Fig. 5**).

Antimicrobial Therapy and Control

Generally, streptococci are sensitive to penicillin and its derivatives, erythromycin, clindamycin, and cephalexin; however, sensitivity testing should be carried out prior to antimicrobial treatment. In endemically affected catteries, vulnerable kittens can be prophylactically treated and the umbilicus dipped in 2% tincture of iodine.[54] Predisposing factors for disease must be minimized.

GGS can be transferred to humans via direct contact and bite wounds. However, the public health risk from *S canis* is low and infection is uncommon, representing 1% of all human streptococcal infections in France over a 5-year period.[61] Serious illness is mainly confined to elderly or immunocompromised patients.

LEPTOSPIRA

Leptospira are fine spiral bacteria (spirochetes), with a central body hooked at each end and surrounded by an envelope. Within this lies a single flagellum arising from each end and overlapping centrally. Species (eg, *L interrogans*) are divided into serovars on the basis of shared envelope antigens.

Leptospirosis occurs in dogs worldwide. The range of serovars reported from each country varies. Reporting depends on (1) those actually present and (2) those sought (which can vary according to the strains used as antigens and the ability of laboratories to isolate and identify them). The dog is a maintenance host of *L interrogans* serovar Canicola, and perhaps of serovar Bratislava.[62] Infection with other serovars is usually sporadic and depends on contact with sources of infection. Serovars present worldwide include Icterohaemorrhagiae and Canicola. Serovars Pomona, Grippotyphosa, and Bratislava are among the most common serovars in North America,[63] with Grippotyphosa and Bratislava the most common in continental Europe.[62]

Infection is transmitted by direct or indirect contact with leptospirae, via ingestion, entry through abrasions, transplacental, and possibly venereal routes. The organisms multiply rapidly to produce a bacteremia, which may cause clinical signs. Leptospirae may cause damage to the liver, kidneys, or other organs; however, the relationship between infecting serovar and organ system involvement is not as well defined as previously thought.[64] Circulating antibody normally limits leptospiremia within 7 to 10 days PI. However, organisms can enter, replicate, and persist in sites protected from circulating antibody, such as renal tissue.[65] Localization may also occur in the pregnant uterus, causing abortion or birth of stillborn or weak progeny.[66,67] Leptospirae may enter the male genital tract from systemic infection.

Clinical Signs

Clinical leptospirosis is rarely recorded in cats,[67] although infection may be common.[68] In dogs, disease of the reproductive tract is uncommon and is associated with systemic infection in most cases (serovars Pomona, Grippotyphosa, and Canicola), and may result from carrier infections (Canicola and Bratislava). Fever and icterus may accompany or precede abortion, or the birth of weak or stillborn progeny. Reproductive disease has been described most consistently in breeding colonies, often associated with serovar Bratislava.[66]

Diagnosis

Diagnosis is confirmed by demonstration of the organism or by the presence of specific antibody. The organisms may be demonstrated by dark ground microscopy of the urine from aborting bitches or in urine, aborted fetuses, or stillborn pups by culture. Dark ground microscopy is relatively insensitive and nonspecific and is no longer recommended.[65] The fragile and fastidious leptospirae may be grown aerobically in complex media, and must be carried out in CL3 facilities to protect laboratory personnel. Primary isolation from tissue or urine takes at least 2 to 6 weeks and is most reliable when the tissue concerned is fresh, uncontaminated, and submitted in a suitable transport medium. Isolation remains the gold standard[63] but is not routinely carried out given that the assay is time-consuming, requires specialist facilities, and may be lacking in sensitivity. The organism, its antigens, or products may also be demonstrated in tissue by silver staining of fixed tissue, by immunofluorescence or immunoperoxidase, and by DNA probes. PCR tests based on sequences from the 16S rRNA gene can also be used to identify the presence of pathogenic leptospirae.[69]

Serologic tests are widely used. Antibodies to leptospirae appear in the serum within 1 to 2 weeks of infection and reach titers of 1:10,000 to 1:30,000 (microscopic agglutination lysis test [MAT]), which may persist for some weeks. The MAT, using live organisms, is the most sensitive test and detects rising titers that follow infection particularly well. ELISAs based on whole cells, axial filaments, and, most specifically, lipoprotein LIPL32 have been described. A competitive ELISA has been produced for serovar Bratislava.[70] Serum antibody can be used to confirm recent infections, but aborting animals or those with reproductive disease may be seronegative. Antibody detected in thoracic exudates from stillborn fetuses is diagnostic. Cross-reaction between serogroups and serovars may occur and accurate serology is best carried out using local serovars.

Antimicrobial Therapy and Control

The parenteral administration of a number of antibiotics such as penicillin, semisynthetic penicillins, streptomycin, and doxycycline is of value in acutely ill animals.

Abortions may be prevented and renal carriers eliminated by doxycycline treatment.[71] Vaccination of uninfected dogs with killed vaccines containing the appropriate serovars prevents reproductive disease. In North America, serovars Pomona, Grippotyphosa, Canicola, and Icterohaemorrhagiae are available in combination. Only serovars Icterohaemorrhagiae and Canicola are available in commercial European vaccines.[62] Infection may be prevented by vaccination, disinfection, elimination of rodents, and restriction of access to rodent-contaminated areas. Leptospirae can survive in uncooked offal and survive freezing, so feeding raw animal byproducts should be avoided.

Humans are a dead-end host for leptospiral infection; contact with the urine or products of abortion of infected dogs should be avoided. Leptospirae enter susceptible hosts via mucous membranes or damaged skin, and gloves and protective clothing should always be worn when handling infected animals. All known shedders or suspected shedders should be treated with antimicrobials to eliminate the carrier state and minimize environmental infectivity. Contaminated areas can be treated with iodophor disinfectants.[65,72]

SALMONELLA

Salmonella spp are gram-negative coliform bacteria. Those causing disease in cats and dogs are serotypes of *S enterica*, especially Typhimurium, Panama, and Montevideo. Salmonellosis is an uncommon cause of reproductive tract disease in the cat and dog and usually follows enteric or systemic disease. Fever or direct bacterial invasion of the products of conception may cause abortion, or the birth of stillborn and weak pups or kittens.[73] *Salmonella* infection can cause prostatitis, orchitis, and epididymitis in males. Cases of *Salmonella* septicemia in greyhound pups can be associated with raw meat diets and a high prevalence of healthy *Salmonella* shedders within racing kennels.[74]

Successful culture confirms infection or carriage. Isolation of salmonellae from organs aseptically sampled from aborted fetuses or stillborn pups or kittens confirms their involvement in reproductive disease.[75] Organisms in feces may be detected by simple PCR, but real-time PCR gives more rapid results. Serum antibody can be detected using ELISA tests based on "O" antigens modified for the dog and cat.

Salmonella may be sensitive in vitro to a wide range of suitable antimicrobials, such as ampicillin, clavulanate-potentiated amoxycillin, gentamicin, or fluoroquinolones, but resistance is common in serotypes such as *S enterica* Typhimurium. Supportive treatment should be given for enteric or systemic signs. *Salmonella* causes clinical disease in humans and protective measures should be taken by those exposed to the products of abortion or to weak puppies or kittens.

CAMPYLOBACTER

Campylobacter spp are microaerobic gram-negative curved rods or short spiral organisms. Up to 14 species have been isolated from dog and cat feces, principally *C jejuni, C coli,* and *C upsaliensis*. Abortion and infection of the female reproductive tract sometimes follow *Campylobacter enteritis,* but are rarely identified in the dog and cat.[76] Infection of the reproductive tract may be ascending or blood-borne; the fetus becomes infected in gravid females, causing abortion or the birth of weak or stillborn pups and kittens. Diagnosis is confirmed by demonstrating the organism in aborted fetuses and vaginal swabs by culture or PCR.[77] Antibody detection is not used routinely in diagnosing infection. Macrolides and fluoroquinolones can be used for treatment. Infection spreads rapidly in multicat or multidog households where

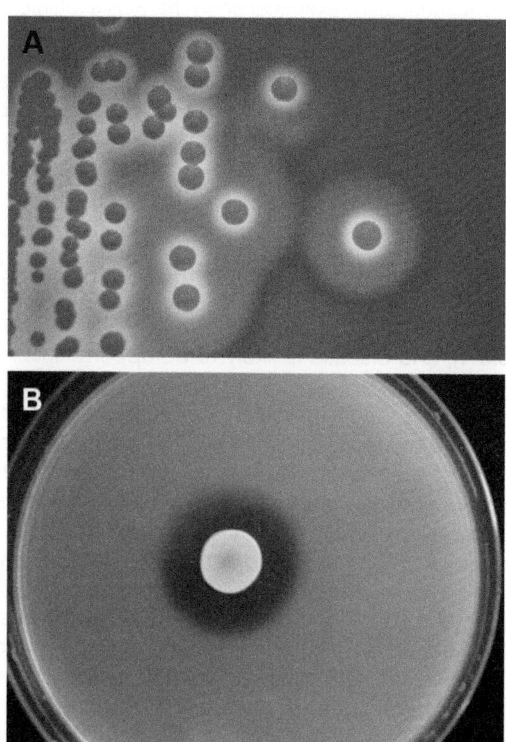

Fig. 6. (*A*) *S pseudintermedius* isolates frequently produce target or double hemolysis on sheep blood agar, a narrow clear zone of hemolysis surrounded by a wide zone of incomplete hemolysis. The ID32 *Staphylococcus* API system can be used to identify *S pseudintermedius*. (*B*) *S pseudintermedius* is DNAse-positive, producing a wide zone of clearing after 24 hours on a DNAse agar plate.

hygiene practice is inadequate. *Campylobacter* spp from cats and dogs can cause disease in humans.

STAPHYLOCOCCUS

Staphylococcus spp contribute to the microflora populating feline and canine skin and mucous membranes. *Staphylococcus pseudintermedius* is the predominant species colonizing canine skin and mucous membranes, and *Staphylococcus felis* is the major species colonizing feline mucous membranes. *S pseudintermedius* is occasionally isolated from feline skin and mucous membranes.

Opportunistic infection of the reproductive tract with staphylococci occurs in the presence of predisposing factors (**Table 2**). Staphylococci are the major cause of mastitis in the bitch and are sporadically recovered from cases of neonatal septicemia, vaginitis, and pyometra.[2,58] A role for *S felis* in feline reproductive disease has yet to be described, but these are significant UTI pathogens[78] and are frequently isolated from other clinical specimens.[79]

Direct microscopy on clinical specimens is useful, with the arrangement of gram-positive cocci in "bunches of grapes." *S pseudintermedius* causes complete or double hemolysis on blood agar (**Fig. 6**) and tests positive on coagulase and DNase tests. *S felis* is weakly hemolytic, coagulase-negative, and weakly DNase-positive[80] and cannot be identified using the commercial ID32 *Staphylococcus* API system. Given the difficulty in distinguishing *S felis* from other staphylococci and that these are coagulase-negative staphylococci, *S felis* infections may be underdiagnosed. Most staphylococcal isolates are susceptible to β-lactamase–resistant synthetic penicillins, first-generation cephalosporins, aminoglycosides, and fluoroquinolones.

MYCOPLASMA

The family Mycoplasmatacaeae contains 3 genera of veterinary significance: *Mycoplasma* spp, *Ureaplasma* spp, and *Acholeplasma* spp, collectively referred to as *Mycoplasma*. Mycoplasmas colonize the epithelial lining of the lower genital tract in cats and dogs (**Table 1**), and disease is likely to be opportunistic.

Experimentally, reproductive disease can be elicited in male and female dogs, and in queens.[81–83] Clinical reproductive disease is occasionally reported but may be underdiagnosed given that mycoplasma culture is not routine in many laboratories. *M canis* was the probable cause of chronic prostatitis and concurrent cystitis in 1 dog, and chronic purulent epididymitis in another.[84] There are few published reports of reproductive disease in cats resulting from natural infection.

Culture is considered the gold standard for diagnosis. However, mycoplasmas have fastidious growth requirements and culture may not be routinely available. Diagnostic laboratories should be consulted prior to sampling to ascertain whether they can carry out the required testing and to request mycoplasma transport medium. The publication of data identifying species-specific sequences has assisted the development of molecular techniques that identify mycoplasmas at both genus and species levels.[85] Mycoplasmas lack rigid cell walls and are inherently resistant to antimicrobial classes that target the cell wall such as the β-lactams. However, mycoplasmas are susceptible to tetracyclines, fluoroquinolones, macrolides and lincosamides.

CHLAMYDOPHILA FELIS

Chlamydophila felis is an obligate intracellular gram-negative organism, which predominantly causes conjunctivitis in cats. Following ocular infection, organisms may spread systemically and persist in many tissues, including the reproductive tract. Cats experimentally infected after 4 months of age shed *C felis* from the reproductive tract within 1 week of ocular infection.[86] Reactivation of shedding may occur in late pregnancy, with the likely spread of infection from the birth canal to kittens via the nasolacrimal ducts.[87] Experimental infection can cause clinical reproductive disease in both queens and toms.[87,88] However, clinical disease caused by natural infection has not been described, and no significant link between reproductive failure and infection has yet been established.[89] A PCR assay to detect the organisms in swabs or tissues is the most sensitive diagnostic test.[90] Prolonged treatment with doxycycline will eliminate conjunctival shedding; persistence in the reproductive tract was not investigated[91] but should be eliminated. Transmission of *C felis* from cats to humans has occasionally been reported.[92]

COXIELLA BURNETII

Coxiella burnetii is an obligate intracellular gram-negative bacterium, the causative agent of query (Q) fever. The organism can infect virtually all animal kingdoms[93] and has a worldwide distribution with the remarkable exception of New Zealand. Infection of cats and dogs may be acquired by tick bites or by ingestion of organisms in infected tissues. The uterus and mammary glands are sites of chronic infection, with recrudescence of shedding during parturition. *C burnetii* was implicated in several cases of abortion and stillbirth in cats, as well as neonatal death in puppies.[94–96] Although all animals were seropositive, in some cases the demonstration of *C burnetii* organisms either was not attempted or was unsuccessful.[95,96] Furthermore, *C burnetii* organisms and DNA have been detected in healthy cat vaginal and uterine tissues[94,97]; therefore, a clear causal relationship cannot be proven. Nonetheless, most reported cases were investigated only because of subsequent disease in humans, and thus *C burnetii*-associated disease in cats and dogs may be underdiagnosed. Because of the zoonotic risk, most cases are diagnosed using serologic methods,[93] although PCR can also be used to demonstrate the organism within tissues. *C burnetii* is sensitive to tetracyclines and fluoroquinolones. Q fever is an important zoonosis worldwide, and seropositive periparturient cats and dogs may provide a source of infection for humans.

LISTERIA MONOCYTOGENES

Listeria monocytogenes is a rare reproductive pathogen in cats and dogs. Clinical disease is usually associated with ingestion of infected meat products. A single report of abortion in a bitch caused by *L monocytogenes* has been published; the bitch presented clinically ill with a brown vaginal discharge 7 weeks into pregnancy, and a pure culture of *L monocytogenes* was isolated from the discharge.[98] Persistent infection of mammary glands can occur, and *L monocytogenes* transmitted in human breast milk caused neonatal death in pups.[99] The organism can be cultured using routine diagnostic media. Individual colonies are surrounded by a wide zone of hemolysis and must be differentiated from βH streptococci. *L monocytogenes* can cause local and systemic disease in humans. *Listeria* is susceptible to aminoglycosides and trimethoprim-sulfonamide.

BARTONELLA

Bartonella spp are intracellular hemotropic gram-negative organisms. The cat is the reservoir host for at least 2 species, *B henselae* and *B clarridgeiae*, and transmission is mainly by athropods. Reproductive failure has been associated with experimental infection in cats although *Bartonella* does not appear to be transmitted transplacentally.[100,101] Establishing a diagnosis is difficult; serology is not always useful since infection is widespread, but a negative result has a high negative predictive value. Bacterial culture is the most reliable diagnostic test, although bacteremia can be intermittent.[102] No antimicrobial protocol has been shown to achieve a long-term cure and antimicrobials should only be used in cats showing clinical signs.[101] Bartonellosis is a significant zoonotic infection.

SUMMARY

Primary exogenous bacterial pathogens, with the exception of *B canis*, are sporadic causes of reproductive disease in the cat and dog. A speculative role for some pathogens such as *C felis*, *C burnetii*, and *Bartonella* spp in reproductive disease has yet to be confirmed. Most bacterial infections of the reproductive tract are caused by endogenous microflora in the presence of predisposing factors, and establishing a definitive diagnosis can be challenging. Bacterial reproductive disease appears to be less significant in the cat, although *Mycoplasma* and *S felis* infections may be underdiagnosed.

ACKNOWLEDGMENTS

We are grateful to Manuel Fuentes and Kathleen Reynolds for generating images for publication.

REFERENCES

1. Clemetson L. Bacterial flora of the vagina and uterus of healthy cats. J Am Vet Med Assoc 1990;196:902–6.
2. Bjurstrom L. Aerobic bacteria occurring in the vagina of bitches with reproductive disorders. Acta Vet Scand 1993;34:29–34.
3. Watts JR, Wright PJ, Whithear KC. Uterine, cervical and vaginal microflora of the normal bitch throughout the reproductive cycle. J Small Anim Pract 1996;37:54–60.
4. Ström Holst B, Bergström A, Lagerstedt A-S, et al. Characterization of the bacterial population of the genital tract of adult cats. Am J Vet Res 2003;64:968.
5. Olson PN, Jones RL, Mather EC. The use and misuse of vaginal cultures in diagnosing reproductive diseases in the bitch. In: Morrow DA, editor. Current therapy in theriogenology. 2nd edition. Philadelphia: WB Saunders; 1986. p. 469–75.
6. Taylor DJ, Renton JP, McGregor AB. Brucella abortus biotype 1 as a cause of abortion in a bitch. Vet Rec 1975;96:428–9.
7. Hinić V, Brodard I, Petridou E, et al. Brucellosis in a dog caused by Brucella melitensis Rev 1. Vet Microbiol 2010;141:391–2.
8. Barr SC, Eilts BE, Roy AF, et al. Brucella suis biotype 1 infection in a dog. J Am Vet Med Assoc 1986;189:686–7.
9. Tolari F, Farina R, Arispici M, et al. Brucellosi nel gatto. Infezione sperimentale con Brucella canis. Ann Sclavo 1982;24:577–85.
10. Repina LP, Nikulina AI, Kosilov IA. Case of brucellosis challenge in humans from a cat. Zh Mikrobiol Epidemiol Immunobiol 1993;4:66–8.
11. Wanke MM. Canine brucellosis. Anim Repro Sci 2004;8283:195–207.
12. Dunne J, Sehgal K, McMillan A, et al. Canine brucellosis In a dog imported into the UK. Vet Rec 2002;151:247.
13. Rittig MG, Alvarez-Martinez MT, Porte F, et al. Intracellular survival of Brucella spp. in human monocytes involves conventional uptake but special phagosomes. Infect Immun 2001;69:3995–4006.
14. Greene CE, Carmichael LE. Canine brucellosis. In: Greene CE, editor. Infectious diseases of the dog and cat. 3rd edition. St Louis (MO): Saunders Elsevier; 2006. p. 369–81.
15. Quinn PJ, Markey BK, Carter ME, et al. Brucella species. In: Quinn PJ, Markey BK, Carter ME, editors. Veterinary microbiology and microbial disease. Oxford (UK): Blackwell Science; 2002. p. 162–7.
16. Kim S, Lee DS, Suzuki H, et al. Detection of Brucella canis and Leptospira interrogans in canine semen by multiplex nested PCR. J Vet Med Sci 2006;68:615–8.
17. Jones LM, Zanardi M, Leong D, et al. Taxonomic position in the genus Brucella of the causative agent of canine abortion. J Bacteriol 1968;95:625–30.
18. Ledbetter EC, Landry MP, Stokol T, et al. Brucella canis endophthalmitis in 3 dogs: clinical features, diagnosis, and treatment. Vet Ophthalmol 2009;12:183–91.
19. Kerwin SC, Lewis DD, Hribernik TN, et al. Diskospondylitis associated with Brucella canis infection in dogs: 14 cases (1980-1991). J Am Vet Med Assoc 1992;201: 1253–7.
20. Carmichael LE, Kenney RM. Canine abortion caused by Brucella canis. J Am Vet Med Assoc 1968;152:605–16.

21. Carmichael LE, Kenney RM. Canine brucellosis: the clinical disease, pathogenesis, and immune response. J Am Vet Med Assoc 1970;156:1726–34.
22. Moore JA, Kakuk TJ. Male dogs natually infected with Brucella canis. J Am Vet Med Assoc 1969;155:1352–8.
23. Schoeb TR, Morton R. Scrotal and testicular changes in canine brucellosis. J Am Vet Med Assoc 1978;172:598–600.
24. Mayer-Scholl A, Draeger A, Göllner C, et al. Advancement of a multiplex PCR for the differentiation of all currently described Brucella species. J Micro Methods 2010;80:112–4.
25. Keid L, Soares R, Vieira N, et al. Diagnosis of canine brucellosis: comparison between serological and microbiological tests and a PCR based on primers to 16S-23S rDNA interspacer. Vet Res Commun 2007;31:951–65.
26. Keid LB, Soares RM, Vasconcellos SA, et al. Comparison of a PCR assay in whole blood and serum specimens for canine brucellosis diagnosis. Vet Rec 2010;167:96–9.
27. Aras Z, Uçan US. Detection of Brucella canis from inguinal lymph nodes of naturally infected dogs by PCR. Theriogenology 2010;74:658–62.
28. Queipo-Ortuno MI, Morata P, Ocon P, et al. Rapid diagnosis of human brucellosis by peripheral-blood PCR assay. J Clin Microbiol 1997;35:2927–30.
29. Carmichael LE, Joubert JC. A rapid slide agglutination test for the serodiagnosis of Brucella canis infection that employs a variant (M–) organism as antigen. Cornell Vet 1987;77:3–12.
30. de Oliveira MZD, Vale V, Keid L, et al. Validation of an ELISA method for the serological diagnosis of canine brucellosis due to Brucella canis. Res Vet Sci 2011;90:425–31.
31. Keid LB, Soares RM, Vasconcellos SA, et al. Comparison of agar gel immunodiffusion test, rapid slide agglutination test, microbiological culture and PCR for the diagnosis of canine brucellosis. Res Vet Sci 2009;86:22–6.
32. Mateu-de-Antonio EM, Martín M. In vitro efficacy of several antimicrobial combinations against Brucella canis and Brucella melitensis strains isolated from dogs. Vet Microbiol 1995;45:1–10.
33. Lawaczeck E, Toporek J, Cwikla J, et al. Brucella canis in a HIV-infected patient. Zoonoses Public Health 2011;58:150–2.
34. Russo TA, Johnson JR. Proposal for a new inclusive designation for extraintestinal pathogenic isolates of Escherichia coli: ExPEC. J Infect Dis 2000;181:1753–4.
35. Wadas B, Kuhn I, Lagerstedt A-S, et al. Biochemical phenotypes of Escherischia coli in dogs: comparison of isolates isolated from bitches suffering from pyometra and urinary tract infection with isolates from faeces of healthy dogs. Vet Microbiol 1996;52:293–300.
36. Siqueira AK, Ribeiro MG, Leite DD, et al. Virulence factors in Escherichia coli strains isolated from urinary tract infection and pyometra cases and from feces of healthy dogs. Res Vet Sci 2009;86:206–10.
37. Barsanti JA. Genitourinary infections. In: Greene CE, editor. Infectious diseases of the dog and cat. 3rd edition. St Louis (MO): Saunders Elsevier; 2006. p. 935–61.
38. Johnston SD, Root Kustritz MV, Olson PNS. Disorders of the canine uterus and uterine tubes. In: Canine and feline theriogenology. Philadelphia: WB Saunders; 2001. p. 206–24.
39. Kenney KJ, Matthiesen DT, Brown NO, et al. Pyometra in cats: 183 cases (1979–1984). J Am Vet Med Assoc 1987;191:1130–2.
40. Sandholm M, Vasenius H, Kivistö A-K. Pathogenesis of canine pyometra. J Am Vet Med Assoc 2011;167:1006–10.

41. Tsumagari S, Ishinazaka T, Kamata H, et al. Induction of canine pyometra by inoculation of Escherichia coli into the uterus and its relationship to reproductive features. Anim Repro Sci 2005;87:301–8.
42. Hagman R, Kühn I. Escherichia coli strains isolated from the uterus and urinary bladder of bitches suffering from pyometra: comparison by restriction enzyme digestion and pulsed-field gel electrophoresis. Vet Microbiol 2002;84:143–53.
43. Linde C. Partial abortion associated with genital Escherichia coli infection in a bitch. Vet Rec 1983;112:454–5.
44. Pretzer SD. Bacterial and protozoal causes of pregnancy loss in the bitch and queen. Theriogenology 2008;70:320–6.
45. Münnich A, Lübke-Becker A. Escherichia coli infections in newborn puppies: clinical and epidemiological investigations. Theriogenology 2004;62:562–75.
46. Normand EH, Gibson NR, Reid SWJ, et al. Antimicrobial-resistance trends in bacterial isolates from companion-animal community practice in the UK. Prev Vet Med 2000;46:267–78.
47. Wedley AL, Maddox TW, Westgarth C, et al. Prevalence of antimicrobial-resistant Escherichia coli in dogs in a cross-sectional, community-based study. Vet Rec 2011;168:354–8.
48. Platell JL, Johnson JR, Cobbold RN, et al. Multidrug-resistant extraintestinal pathogenic Escherichia coli of sequence type ST131 in animals and foods. Vet Microbiol 2011. [Epub ahead of print].
49. Vela AI, Falsen E, Simarro I, et al. Neonatal mortality in puppies due to bacteremia by Streptococcus dysgalactiae subsp. dysgalactiae. J Clin Microbiol 2006;44:666–8.
50. Dow SW, Jones RL, Thomas TN, et al. Group B streptococcal infection in two cats. J Am Vet Med Assoc 1987;190:71–2.
51. Kornblatt AN, Adams RL, Barthold SW, et al. Canine neonatal deaths associated with group B streptococcal septicaemia. J Am Vet Med Assoc 1983;183:700–1.
52. Mantovani A, Restani R, Sciarra D, et al. Streptococcus L infection in the dog. J Small Anim Pract 1961;2:185–94.
53. Davies ME, Skulski G. A study of beta-haemolytic streptococci in the fading puppy in relation to canine virus hepatitis in the dam. Br Vet J 1956;112:404–15.
54. Greene CE, Prescott JF. Streptococcal and other gram-positive bacterial infections. In: Greene CE, editor. Infectious diseases of the dog and cat. 3rd edition. St Louis (MO): Saunders Elsevier; 2006. p. 302–16.
55. Johnson C. Diagnosis and treatment of chronic vaginitis in the bitch. Vet Clin North Am Small Anim Pract 1991;21.3:523–31.
56. Jung C, Wehrend A, Konig A, et al. Investigations about the incidence, differentiation and microbiology of canine mastitis. Praktische Tierarzt 2002;86:508–11.
57. Gruffydd-Jones TJ. Acute mastitis in a cat. Feline Pract 1980;10:41–2.
58. Schäfer-Somi S, Spergser J, Breitenfellner J, et al. Bacteriological status of canine milk and septicaemia in neonatal puppies: a retrospective study. J Vet Med 2003; 50:343–6.
59. Lamm CG, Ferguson AC, Lehenbauer TW, et al. Streptococcal infection in dogs. Vet Pathol 2010;47:387–95.
60. Quinn PJ, Carter ME, Markey BK, et al. The streptococci and related cocci. In: Quinn PJ, Markey BK, Carter ME, editor. Clinical veterinary microbiology. London: Wolfe; 1994. p. 127–36.
61. Galpérine T, Cazorla C, Blanchard E, et al. Streptococcus canis infections in humans: retrospective study of 54 patients. J Infect 2007;55:23–6.
62. Ellis WA. Control of canine leptospirosis in Europe. Vet Rec 2010;167:602–5.

63. Goldstein RE. Canine leptospirosis. Vet Clin North Am Small Anim Pract 2010;40: 1091–101.
64. Goldstein RE, Lin RC, Langston CE, et al. Influence of infecting serogroup on clinical features of leptospirosis in dogs. J Vet Intern Med 2006;20:489–94.
65. Greene CE, Sykes JE, Brown CA, et al. Leptospirosis. In: Greene CE, editor. Infectious diseases of the dog and cat. 3rd edition. St Louis (MO): Saunders Elsevier; 2006. p. 402–17.
66. Ellis WA. Leptospirosis. J Small Anim Pract 1986;27:683–92.
67. Reilly GAC, Baillie NC, Morrow WT, et al. Feline stillbirths associated with mixed Salmonella typhimurium and leptospira infection. Vet Rec 1994;135:608.
68. Andre-Fontaine G. Canine leptospirosis: do we have a problem? Vet Microbiol 2006;117:19–24.
69. Fearnley C, Wakely PR, Gallego-Beltran J, et al. The development of a real-time PCR to detect pathogenic Leptospira species in kidney tissue. Res Vet Sci 2011;85:8–16.
70. Frizzell C, Mackie DP, Montgomery JM, et al. Development of a competitive ELISA for the detection of serum antibodies of Leptospira serovar Bratislava. Pig J 2004; 53:195–9.
71. Langston CE, Heuter KJ. Leptospirosis. A re-emerging zoonotic disease. Vet Clin North Am Small Anim Pract 2003;33:791–807.
72. Van de Maele I, Claus A, Haesebrouck F, et al. Leptospirosis in dogs: a review with emphasis on clinical aspects. Vet Rec 2011;163:409–13.
73. Caldow GL, Graham MM. Abortion in foxhounds and a ewe flock associated with Salmonella montevideo infection. Vet Rec 1998;142:138–9.
74. Morley PS, Strohmeyer R, Tankson JD, et al. Evaluation of the association between feeding raw meat and Salmonella enterica infections at a greyhound breeding facility. J Am Vet Med Assoc 2006;228:1524–32.
75. Reilly GAC, Baillie NC, Morrow WT, et al. Feline stillbirths associated with mixed Salmonella typhimurium and leptospira infection. Vet Rec 1994;135:608.
76. Bulgin MS, Ward AC, Sriranganathan N, et al. Abortion in the dog due to Campylobacter species. Am J Vet Res 1984;45:556.
77. Chaban B, Musil KM, Himsworth CG, et al. Development of CPN-based real-time quantitative PCR assays for the detection of 14 Campylobacter species and application to screening of canine faecal samples. Appl Environ Microbiol 2009;75:3055–61.
78. Litster A, Moss SM, Honnery M, et al. Prevalence of bacterial species in cats with clinical signs of lower urinary tract disease: recognition of Staphylococcus felis as a possible feline urinary tract pathogen. Vet Microbiol 2007;121:188.
79. Igimi S, Atobe H, Tohya Y, et al. Characterization of the most frequent encountered Staphylococcus sp in cats. Vet Microbiol 1994;39:260.
80. Igimi S, Kawamura S, Takahashi E, et al. Staphylococcus felis, a new species from clinical specimens from cats. Int J Syst Bacteriol 1989;39:373–7.
81. Holzmann A, Laber G, Walzl H. Experimentally induced mycoplasma infection in the genital tract of the female dog. Theriogenology 1979;12:355–70.
82. Tan RJS, Miles JA. Incidence and significance of mycoplasmas in sick cats. Res Vet Sci 1974;16:27–34.
83. Laber G, Holzmann A. Experimentally induced mycoplasmal infection in the genital tract of the male dog. Theriogenology 1977;7:177–88.
84. L'Abee-Lund TM, Heiene R, Friis NF, et al. Mycoplasma canis and urogenital disease in dogs in Norway. Vet Rec 2003;153:235.
85. Chalker VJ, Brownlie J. Taxonomy of the canine Mollicutes by 16S rRNA gene and 16S/23S rRNA intergenic spacer region sequence comparison. Int J Syst Evol Microbiol 2004;54:537–42.

86. TerWee J, Sabara M, Kokjohn K, et al. Characterization of the systemic disease and ocular signs induced by experimental infection with Chlamydia psittaci in cats. Vet Microbiol 1998;59:259–81.
87. Greene CE. Chlamydial infections. In: Greene CE, editor. Infectious diseases of the dog and cat. 3rd edition. St Louis (MO): Saunders Elsevier; 2006. p. 245–52.
88. Kane JL, Woodland RM, Elder MG, et al. Chlamydial pelvic infection in cats: a model for the study of human pelvic inflammatory disease. Genitourin Med 1985;61:311–8.
89. Sykes JE, Anderson GA, Studdert VP, et al. Prevalence of feline Chlamydia psittaci and feline herpesvirus 1 in cats with upper respiratory tract disease. J Vet Intern Med 1999;13:153–62.
90. McDonald M, Willett BJ, Jarrett O, et al. A comparison of DNA amplification, isolation and serology for the detection of Chlamydia psittaci infection in cats. Vet Rec 1998;143:97–101.
91. Dean R, Harley R, Helps C, et al. Use of quantitative real-time PCR to monitor the response of Chlamydophila felis infection to doxycycline treatment. J Clin Microbiol 2005;43:1858–64.
92. Hartley JC, Stevenson S, Robinson AJ, et al. Conjunctivitis due to Chlamydophila felis (Chlamydia psittaci feline pneumonitis agent) acquired from a cat: case report with molecular characterization of isolates from the patient and cat. J Infect 2001; 43:7–11.
93. Maurin M, Raoult D. Q fever. Clin Microbiol Rev 2011;12:518–53.
94. Nagaoka H, Sugieda M, Akiyama M, et al. Isolation of Coxiella burnettii from the vagina of feline clients at veterinary clinics. J Vet Med Sci 1998;60:251–2.
95. Marrie TJ, MacDonald A, Durant H, et al. An outbreak of Q fever probably due to contact with a parturient cat. Chest 1988;93:98–103.
96. Buhariwalla F, Cann B, Marrie TJ. A dog-related outbreak of Q fever. Clin Infect Dis 1996;23:753–5.
97. Cairns K, Brewer M, Lappin MR. Prevalence of Coxiella burnetii DNA in vaginal and uterine samples from healthy cats of north-central Colorado. J Feline Med Surg 2007;9:196–201.
98. Sturgess CP. Listerial abortion in the bitch. Vet Rec 1989;124:177.
99. Svabic-Vlahovic V, Pantic D, Pavicic M. Transmission of Listeria monocytogenes from mother's milk to her baby and to puppies. Lancet 1988;2:1201.
100. Guptill L, Slater LN, Wu CC, et al. Evidence of reproductive failure and lack of perinatal transmission of Bartonella henselae in experimentally infected cats. Vet Immunol Immunopath 1998;65:177–89.
101. Guptill-Yoran L. Bartonellosis. In: Greene CE, editor. Infectious diseases of the dog and cat. 3rd edition. St Louis (MO): Saunders Elsevier; 2006. p. 510–24.
102. Abbott RC, Chomel BB, Kasten RW, et al. Experimental and natural infection with Bartonella henselae in domestic cats. Comp Immunol Micro Infect Dis 1997;20:41–51.
103. Tan RJS, Lim EW, Ishak B. Ecology of Mycoplasmas in clinically healthy cats. Aust Vet J 1977;53:515–8.
104. Ling GV, Ruby AL. Aerobic bacterial flora of the prepuce, urethra, and vagina of normal adult dogs. Am J Vet Res 1978;39:695–8.
105. Olson PNS, Mather EC. Canine vaginal and uterine bacterial flora. J Am Vet Med Assoc 1978;172:708–11.
106. Johnston SD, Root Kustritz MV, Olson PNS. The neonate: from birth to weaning. In: Canine and feline theriogenology. Philadelphia: WB Saunders; 2001. p. 146–67.

Viral Reproductive Pathogens of Dogs and Cats

Nicola Decaro, DVM, PhD[a], Leland E. Carmichael, DVM[b], Canio Buonavoglia, DVM[a,*]

KEYWORDS

• Viruses • Dogs • Cats • Reproductive pathogens

Viruses represent a significant cause of reproductive failures in both dogs and cats. Pregnancy losses can be caused by transplacental transmission of virus with direct infection of embryos and fetuses or, less frequently, by severe debilitation of pregnant animals in the absence of congenital infection.[1] In addition to the direct effect on pregnancy, certain viruses, such as the minute virus of canines (MVC), canine herpesvirus (CaHV), and feline panleukopenia virus (FPLV), can cause perinatal infections leading to neonatal mortality or abnormalities.[2–4] This review discusses viral infections that affect canine and feline pregnancy, with particular emphasis on pathologic, diagnostic, and prophylactic features.

CANINE VIRAL REPRODUCTIVE PATHOGENS

Canid Herpesvirus 1

Canid herpesvirus 1 (CaHV-1) is an alphaherpevirus closely related to felid herpesvirus 1, phocid herpesvirus 1, and equid herpesviruses 1 and 4.[5] Only dogs are fully susceptible to CaHV-1 infection and disease, although specific antibodies have been found in wild carnivores worldwide. By serologic investigations, the virus has been shown to be widespread in domestic dog populations, with the highest seroprevalence in kenneled dogs. Virus transmission usually occurs through direct contact with genital or oronasal secretion of infected animals. The clinical course of CaHV-1 infection depends on the age of infected pups, with the fatal, systemic form of disease occurring in puppies less than 2 weeks of age.[3] In fact, CaHV-1 replicates best at temperatures lower than 36°C (96.8°F), which are commonly observed in the first week after birth. Newborn puppies can be infected during passage through the birth

The authors have nothing to disclose.

[a] Department of Veterinary Public Health, Faculty of Veterinary Medicine of Bari, Strada per Casamassima Km 3, 70010 Valenzano, Bari, Italy
[b] James A. Baker Institute for Animal Health, Cornell University, Ithaca, NY 14853, USA
* Corresponding author.
E-mail address: c.buonavoglia@veterinaria.uniba.it

Vet Clin Small Anim 42 (2012) 583–598
doi:10.1016/j.cvsm.2012.01.006 vetsmall.theclinics.com

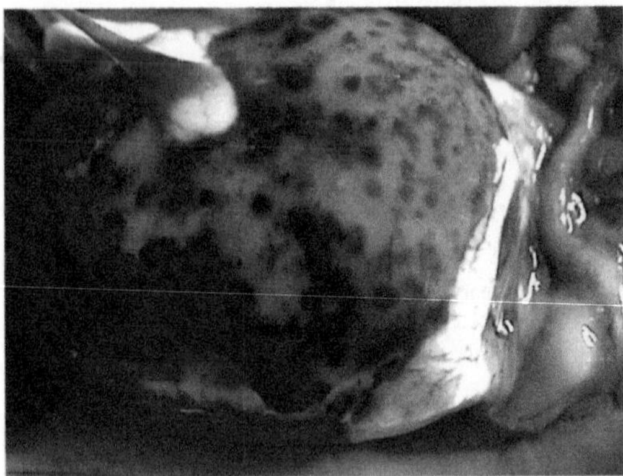

Fig. 1. Puppy with natural neonatal CaHV-1 infection. Multiple renal hemorrhages are evident.

canal or by contact with oronasal secretions of infected animals. CaHV-1–induced generalized disease is characterized by loss of appetite, abdominal pain, soft feces or diarrhea, ataxia, serosanguineous nasal discharge, and mucosal hemorrhages. The death of infected puppies usually occurs at 3 to 7 days after the appearance of clinical signs and may involve an entire litter. Although puppies older than 2 weeks usually develop subclinical disease, neurologic disorders have been associated to CaHV-1 infection.[6]

In neonates that die as a consequence of systemic infections, postmortem findings are pathognomonic, consisting of scattered hemorrhages within the kidney (**Fig. 1**), multifocal areas of necrosis in the liver and lungs, and enlargement of spleen and lymph nodes. Histologically, the prevalent lesions are represented by foci of hemorrhage and necrosis with eosinophilic intranuclear viral inclusions in parenchymatous organs.[7]

CaHV-1 is uncommonly associated with transplacental infections, leading to fetal or neonatal death. The effects of in utero infection depend of the age of gestation when infection occurs. Bitches infected at mid-gestation may abort or deliver stillborn puppies in the absence of other clinical signs including vaginal discharge. Some puppies may appear normal but develop the systemic form within few days after birth.[8] After in utero infection, multifocal necrotizing lesions are evident in the placentas, whereas findings in aborted fetuses are similar to those observed in the systemic neonatal form. The uterus of infected bitches may contain dead fetuses of varied sizes (**Fig. 2**).

In adult dogs, CaHV-1 is believed to be responsible for infectious tracheobronchitis, but it has not proved to be a primary agent. Canine infectious respiratory disease (CIRD) is multifactorial and may be caused by several viruses (CaHV-1, canine adenoviruses, canine coronavirus, canine distemper virus, canine parainfluenza virus, canine influenza virus) and bacteria (*Bordetella bronchispetica*, *Mycoplasma* spp, *Streptococcus* spp).[9] However, sexually mature dogs may develop venereal infections characterized by lymphofollicular (**Fig. 3**) and/or papulovesicular lesions and hyperemia of the genital tract.

Gross lesions of puppies affected with CaHV-1 infection are usually diagnostic; histopathology can be performed for confirmation. Diagnosis of CaHV-1 infection can also be obtained by virus isolation on susceptible cell lines of canine origin, immunofluorescence assay on tissue sections or smears, and the polymerase chain reaction (PCR). Recently, a real-time PCR assay, based on the TaqMan technology,

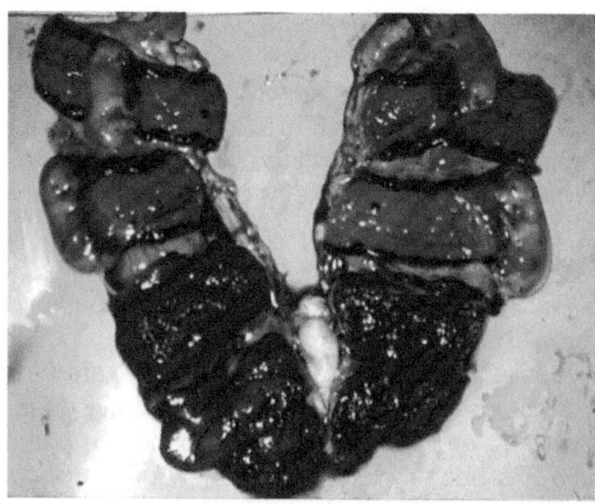

Fig. 2. Uterus of pregnant bitch with experimental CaHV-1 infection. The fetuses are of various sizes and stages of decomposition. (*Courtesy of* Dr A. Hashimoto, Hokkaido University, Japan.)

has been developed for detection and quantification of CaHV-1 DNA.[10] Clinical samples suitable for CaHV-1 diagnosis include kidney or other affected organs from dead neonates or aborted fetuses, nasal and pharyngeal swabs from CIRD-affected dogs, and vaginal or preputial swabs from adult dogs with lesions in the genital tract. Serology, using immunofluorescence or virus neutralization, may help assess virus circulation in kennels and rescue shelters, but it is not the gold standard for diagnosis of active infections due to the propensity of CaHV-1 to establish latency.

To date, there is no effective treatment for CaHV-1 neonatal infections. Experimental elevation of the environmental temperature resulted in suppressed viral replication, but it is ineffective as a treatment.[11] Administration of antiviral drugs (eg, vidarabine or acyclovir) has been shown to be effective against human herpesviruses, but trials

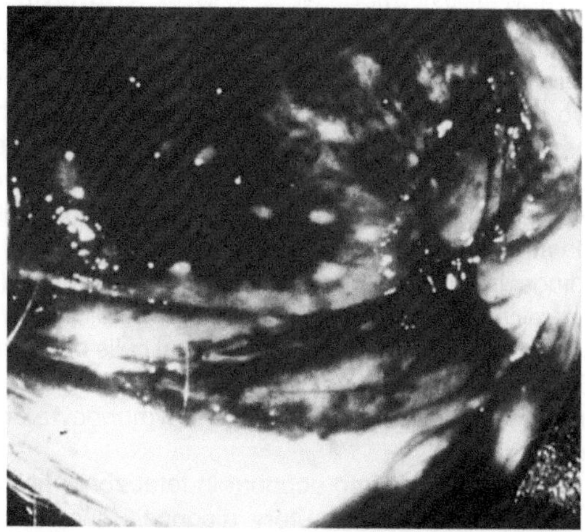

Fig. 3. Bitch with natural CaHV-1 infection. The vaginal mucosa is multifocally hemorrhagic. (*Courtesy of* Dr A. Hashimoto, Hokkaido University, Japan.)

in dogs have not produced conclusive results.[7] CaHV-1 vaccination may be used in breeding kennels with reproductive disorders to immunize bitches before mating in order to protect pregnancy and prevent infection of newborns. In Europe, a subunit vaccine containing CaHV-1 glycoprotein B is available, although its efficacy has been questioned. This vaccine should be administered only to bitches during heat or in the early pregnancy and again at 6 to 7 weeks of gestation.[3]

Canine Minute Virus (Canine Parvovirus 1)

Canine minute virus (CnMV), also known as MVC or canine parvovirus type 1 (CPV-1), was first isolated from the feces of asymptomatic dogs in 1967.[12] CnMV is an autonomous parvovirus genetically and antigenically unrelated to canine parvovirus type 2 (CPV-2), which causes fatal gastroenteritis in young dogs.[13] Recent studies have shown that CnMV is more closely related to bovine parvovirus and human bocaviruses, and now has been included in the new genus *Bocavirus* of the family Parvoviridae.[14] Only dogs have been shown to be susceptible to CnMV infection. Serologic investigations have demonstrated seroprevalences of 5% to 15.4% in Japan, 5.6% in Germany, 11.8% in Korea, 13.6% to 17.6% in Italy, 18% in Turkey, and 30% to 70% in the United States.[4,15]

CnMV infection has been associated with a variety of clinical forms, including asymptomatic infections, respiratory distress, enteric disease, neonatal mortality, and reproductive disorders.[4] The virus has been detected by virus isolation or PCR in the feces of both healthy and diarrheic dogs.[12,16] Experimental infections of puppies of different ages with the original isolate of Binn[12] that had been passaged several times in cell culture failed to reproduce the disease, but the virus was recovered from the feces and internal organs of inoculated pups.[17] In a subsequent experiment with a low-passage CnMV isolate,[18] 5-day-old puppies had severe respiratory, but not enteric disease. Natural outbreaks of CnMV-associated neonatal mortality have been reported.[18–21] Puppies infected at less than 4 weeks of age often had mild or vague symptoms preceding their rapid death; others displayed depression, loss of appetite, acute myocarditis, respiratory distress, and/or enteritis.[4] Virus-induced immunosuppression due to reduction of monocyte phagocytosis may play a role in CnVM pathogenesis.[22]

Analogous to other parvoviruses, CnMV can cause transplacental infections leading to subclinical disease, embryonic resorption, abortion, birth deformities, or neonatal mortality.[4] Different outcomes of CnMV infection in pregnant bitches depend on the time of infection during gestation. Infections during the first half of pregnancy may result in embryo death and resorption (**Fig. 4**), whereas stillbirths and the birth of weak pups are more frequently observed in the late stages of pregnancy.[18] Direct inoculation of fetuses in late gestation resulted in arrested fetal development (**Fig. 5**). Recently, CnMV was reported to be associated with neurologic disease in dogs of various ages[23] and with severe gastroenteritis in an elderly dog.[24]

Postmortem findings in nursing puppies include pneumonia (**Fig. 6**), enteritis, myocarditis, and thymic edema and atrophy. Histopathologically, eosinophilic intranuclear viral inclusions are observed in the epithelial cells of intestinal crypts and in myocardiocytes. Other histologic changes are hyperplasia of the intestinal crypts, necrosis of myocardium, interstitial pneumonia, and lymphocyte depletion in thymus and other lymphoid tissues.[4]

CnMV infection should be taken into account in fetal abnormalities, abortion, and neonatal mortality. Samples for a laboratory diagnosis should consist of fetal or neonatal tissues such as myocardium, intestine, and lungs. CnMV diagnosis is based on virus isolation on Walter Reed canine cells (3873D cells), followed by detection of

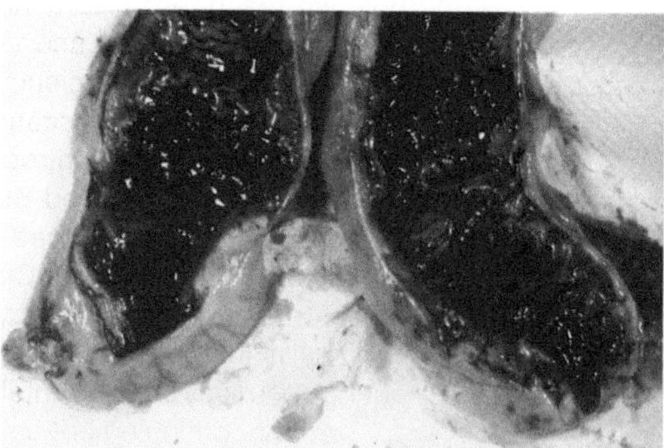

Fig. 4. Uterus from a bitch with experimental CnMV infection (early gestation). There is embryo death, decomposition, and resorption.

intranuclear inclusion bodies by hematoxylin-eosin staining or of viral antigens by immunofluorescence, using specific antibodies. Recently, Madin-Darby canine kidney cells also have been shown to support viral replication in vitro. In addition, PCR protocols are available for sensitive and rapid detection of viral nucleic acid.[16]

As with most viral infection, there is no effective treatment for CnMV infections due to the rapid progression of disease. Vaccines are not available since the full impact of CnMV on canine health is unknown.[15]

Bluetongue Virus

Bluetongue is a noncontagious viral disease of domestic and certain wild ruminants caused by bluetongue virus (BTV), a member of the genus *Orbivirus* within family Reoviridae. Clinical evidence of BTV infection has been reported in sheep, some wild ruminants and, rarely, cattle. Multiple BTV serotypes and strains can colonize the pregnant uterus and, subsequently, the embryo and fetus. Reproductive failures occur in

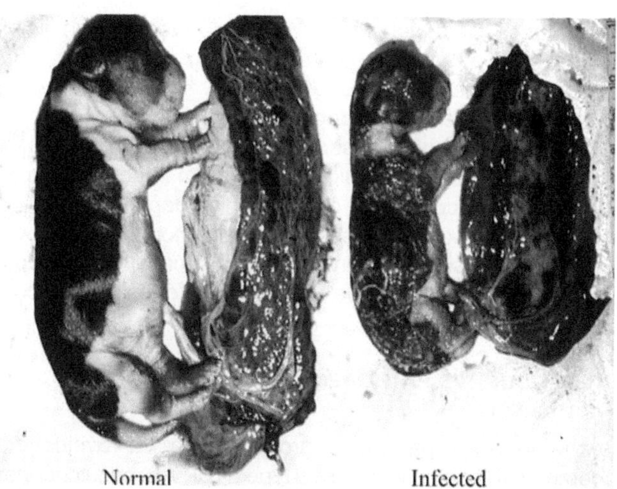

Fig. 5. Canine fetus (*right*) with experimental CnMV infection (late gestation). There is arrested fetal development in comparison to an uninfected puppy (*left*).

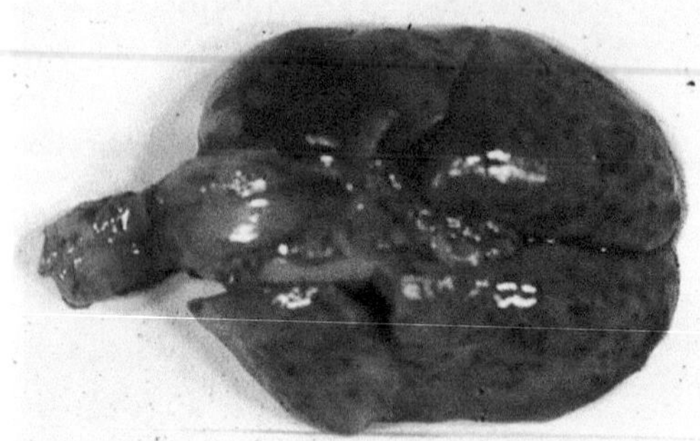

Fig. 6. Lung from a puppy with experimental CnMV neonatal infection. There are scattered areas of hemorrhage.

both pregnant sheep and cattle and include early embryonic death, abortion, and fetal malformations. Bulls and rams may be affected by temporary sterility or infertility.[25]

Bluetongue was reported in dogs in the United States that were given a multivalent canine vaccine contaminated by a BTV-11 strain.[26,27] The source appeared to be contaminated fetal calf serum that was used for cell propagation. This virus was responsible for abortion and/or death in late-term pregnant bitches, whereas non-pregnant dogs had only subclinical infections and seroconversion. The affected pregnant bitches presented with depression and fever within 2 to 3 days after vaccination and abortion few days later. Some of them developed severe respiratory distress and either died or were euthanatized. At necropsy, the animals appeared normal or displayed moderate gross lesions, mainly moderate to severe pulmonary edema. Postmortem findings similar to those commonly observed in BTV-infected sheep were present only in one case and included sanguineous pleural effusion, serous pericardial fluid, hemorrhagic areas in the lungs, and degenerated kidneys. Histopathology revealed pulmonary edema and congestion and placental vasculitis in all cases, with degenerative cardiomyopathy, diffuse glomerulonephropathy, and centrolobular hepatocellular degeneration being reported only in one bitch. These findings were confirmed by experimental inoculation of pregnant bitches with the contaminated vaccine or the isolated BTV-11 strain.[28,29]

For prevention of BTV infection in dogs, fetal calf serum and all bovine-derived products to be used in dogs should be screened for the presence of BTV.[25,26] Nothing is currently known about the transmission of BTV from infected dogs to susceptible ruminants. However, the occurrence of viremia in dogs that were administered contaminated vaccines[26,27] or those experimentally inoculated,[28,29] as well as the circulation of several BTV serotypes in African wild carnivores,[30] poses concerns about the potential epidemiologic role of domestic dogs in the context of BTV outbreaks involving ruminants.

FELINE VIRAL REPRODUCTIVE PATHOGENS

Feline Panleukopenia Virus

FPLV belongs to the feline parvovirus group of the Parvoviridae family (genus *Parvovirus*), together with canine parvovirus type 2 (CPV-2) and other parvoviruses of carnivores. FPLV-induced disease in cats has been known since the beginning of the 20th century, whereas CPV-2 emerged as pathogens of dogs only in the late 1970s.[31]

FPLV has maintained genetic stability,[32] whereas CPV-2 has experienced higher rates of nucleotide changes.[33,34] Within a few years after its first emergence, the "original" CPV-2 (1978 isolates) was completely replaced by 2 antigenic variants: CPV-2a and CPV-2b. A third antigenic variant (CPV-2c) was detected in Italy in 2000.[35] The latter variant is now spreading efficiently in the canine population worldwide.[31] CPV antigenic variants differ from the original type 2 by amino acid changes affecting the capsid protein and by their extended host range, which includes canine and feline cells in vitro and dogs and cats in vivo.[36] In fact, CPV-2a, CPV-2b, and CPV-2c viruses have been isolated from cats with clinical signs of feline panleukopenia.[37–41] Although CPV-2 has been tentatively associated with congenital cerebellar hypoplasia in pups, it is not recognized as a primary cause of reproductive failures in dogs. However, due to the expanded host range to cats, this virus might cause congenital infection in the feline species.

FPLV is shed in high amounts in the feces of infected cats. The virus, transmitted by the fecal-oral route, replicates in lymphoid tissues associated with the oropharynx, spreading to mitotically active tissues by both a cell-free and leukocyte-associated viremia. Target tissues include lymphoid organs, bone marrow, intestinal crypts, and, in pregnant queens, fetuses.[2,42] The clinical course and outcome of FPLV infection depend on the time when this is acquired (prenatal or postnatal). Postnatal infections of 2- to 6-month-old kittens result in the classic form of feline panleukopenia, characterized by fever, loss of appetite, depression, haemorrhagic diarrhoea, vomiting, and dehydration. A profound leukopenia involving all white blood cell (WBC) populations is constantly observed, with WBC counts ranging from 50 to 3000 cells/μL.[2] Intrauterine infections can cause different reproductive disorders that vary according to the stage of pregnancy at the moment of infection. Early in utero infections commonly result in infertility, early fetal death, and resorption, whereas in mid-gestation abortion or fetal mummification is more frequent. Queens that suffer abortion may not develop other clinical signs.

In the late stage of pregnancy, FPLV invades fetal nervous tissues, including the cerebrum, cerebellum, optic nerve, and retina. Virus-induced lesions are represented by hydrocephalus, hydranencephaly, cerebellar hypoplasia, optic nerve atrophy, and retinopathy. The cerebellum is the most damaged tissue, because, in cats, this part of central nervous system develops during late gestation and early neonatal periods.[43,44] The same lesions also may be observed when infection occurs within 10 days after birth. Cerebellar hypoplasia in FPLV-infected neonatal kittens is a consequence of Purkinje cell degeneration and interference with cortical development.[45,46] Newborn kittens with neurologic disorders due to FPLV perinatal infection often display tremors and incoordination due to the cerebellar injury and other neurologic disorders (seizures, behavioral changes) as a result of the forebrain damage. Retinal degeneration and optic nerve atrophy may lead to a certain degree of blindness. Gross pathologic changes in postnatal infections consist of hemorrhagic enteritis and lymphoadenopathy, which are characterized at the microscopic level by necrosis of the crypts and shortening of the villi in the intestine and by lymphocyte depletion in all lymphoid tissues. In utero infected kittens may have a spectrum of neurologic lesions (cerebellar hypoplasia, hydranencephaly, hydrocephalus) and thymic atrophy. Histologically, the most prominent change is the disruption of normal cerebellar architecture, with marked reduction of the granular and Purkinje cell layers. Vacuolation of the parenchyma, astrocytosis, and disruption of ependymal cells are also observed in the cerebrum of prenatally infected kittens.

A rapid diagnosis of FPLV infection is especially important in multicat households in order to isolate infected cats and prevent secondary infections of susceptible contact animals. The clinical diagnosis of feline panleukopenia is inconclusive and it should be always confirmed by laboratory tests. Several methods have been developed for the laboratory diagnosis, which can be carried out on the faces or intestinal contents and on nervous tissues in postnatal and prenatal infections, respectively. Parvovirus infection in cats is diagnosed by means of immunochromatographic tests, virus isolation on feline cells, hemagglutination (HA), and PCR, but none of these methods is able to differentiate FPLV from CPV. Virus isolation on cell lines of different origin, hemagglutination inhibition (HI) tests with monoclonal antibodies (MAbs), or sequence analysis of large fragments of the main capsid protein VP2 gene can discriminate between the feline and canine parvoviruses, but they are not always applicable. Minor groove binder (MGB) probe assays have been used successfully for prediction of the CPV type in the dog feces,[47,48] as well as for discrimination between vaccinal and field strains of CPV,[49,50] even when these viruses are present simultaneously in the same samples.[51] An MGB assay also has been established for detection of FPLV and its rapid discrimination from CPV-2.[52]

Supportive therapy and nursing care reduce FPLV-associated mortality. In postnatal infections, parental fluid therapy is recommended to restore fluid, electrolytic, and acid-base balance. Restriction of oral intake of water and food is needed if vomiting persists and parenteral administration of broad-spectrum antibiotics may help prevent bacterial secondary infections. Antiviral therapy using feline recombinant interferon-omega has had variable efficacy in dogs with CPV-induced enteritis, but there are no data regarding the feline host.[42] There is no adequate treatment for neonatal kittens with FPLV-induced neurologic disorders.

Strict isolation is indicated when a cat is diagnosed with FPLV infection. The most effective prophylactic measure against FPLV infection is vaccination of susceptible cats. Both killed and modified-live virus (MLV) vaccines are available, but the latter are most effective and have been shown to provide protection for at least 6 years. The primary causes of FPLV vaccination failures are interfering levels of MDA that are transmitted by queens to their offspring through colostrum. Thus, in order to avoid interference with active immunization, vaccines should be administered to kittens only after MDA have waned.[42] In addition, MLV FPLV vaccines should never be administered to kittens less than 4 weeks of age to avoid cerebellar damage or to pregnant queens. Although some killed vaccines are licensed for use in pregnant queens, the value of vaccination is questionable and should be avoided.

There are concerns about the efficacy of FPLV-based vaccines against the CPV-2 antigenic variants. In a recent study,[53] an FPV-based vaccine protected against subsequent infection with a virulent CPV-2b strain. In that study, however, only 2 vaccinated cats were used, and they were challenged shortly after the administration of the second vaccine dose. Additional studies are required to confirm those findings, but the development of multivalent vaccines containing FPV in combination with a CPV variant strain might be considered.[40,41]

Feline Immunodeficiency Virus

Feline immunodeficiency virus (FIV) is a retrovirus of the genus *Lentivirus* that shares pathobiological features with human immunodeficiency virus (HIV). Although first identified only in 1986, FIV is now recognized as an endemic pathogen in the domestic cat populations worldwide, reaching a prevalence of 28% in some countries.[54] To date, at least 5 genetically distinct subtypes or clades have been defined according to the sequence diversity of the *env* gene, with clades A and B including most strains detected in the field.[55]

FIV transmission from infected to healthy cats occurs mainly by parental inoculation of free virus or virus-infected leukocytes through bite wounds, accounting for the higher prevalence in free-ranging intact male cats. Virus transmission from infected queens to their kittens is sporadically observed under natural conditions, but it is constantly reproduced in experimental infections. Vertical transmission also may occur in utero via the transplacental route, during parturition through direct contact with the genital secretions, or postpartum through ingestion of infected colostrum or milk. Milk has been shown to contain high concentrations of virus, which also occurs in mammary gland tissue. Not all kittens of the same litter become FIV infected. However, the high FIV-induced mortality, or progressive disease, in kittens born to FIV-positive queens observed under experimental infections suggests a higher frequency of natural in utero and neonatal infections than previously believed. Vertical transmission is more efficient when pregnant queens are infected during gestation. An increased rate of FIV infection with the advancement of pregnancy has been demonstrated. It was found that fetuses from cats infected with FIV at 3 weeks of gestation did not become infected, but up to 60% were found to be virus positive when queens were infected later in pregnancy.[56]

Transmission of virus between cats in stable households is uncommon.[57] Infected cats may remain healthy for several years before they develop disease signs and some cats never develop disease. The clinical course of FIV infection classically follows 3 stages: an acute phase of infection characterized by mild clinical signs (lethargy, fever, anorexia, lymphoadenopathy), a long-term asymptomatic phase, and a final phase, known as "acquired immunodeficiency syndrome–related complex." Typical signs of this phase are chronic gingivostomatitis, rhinitis and enteritis, lymphoadenopathy, weight loss, immune-mediated glomerulonephritis, neurologic disorders, and neoplasms. Also, secondary infections by opportunistic pathogens may occur.[57,58]

FIV infection may contribute to aberrant pregnancies and reproduction failures, resulting in arrested fetal development, abortion, stillbirth, and lowered birth weights.[59] A high rate of stillbirths or neonatal deaths has been observed in kittens born to FIV-infected queens, especially if infection had been acquired early in pregnancy.[56,60] Although data concerning fetal viability differ, an increased number of nonviable kittens, either due to arrested development or fetal resorption, has been reported in experimentally infected queens compared with uninfected queens.[61,62] The average birth weights and postnatal weight gains of FIV-infected kittens were generally lower than those of kittens born to uninfected queens, even in the absence of vertical transmission.[61] A different FIV distribution in fetal tissues has been detected according to the viral strain.[56,60]

Diagnostic tests for FIV are based on the detection of antibodies against the structural proteins (capsid protein p24 or transmembrane peptides) by in-house ELISA or immunochromatographic tests. Since young kittens born to FIV-infected queens may test falsely positive, due to the presence of MDA, they should be retested at 16 weeks of age. In addition, false-negative results may be related to the lack of seroconversion in the early stage of infection and to the immunodeficiency induced in the late stage of infection. In those cases, direct methods, such as PCR and real-time PCR, can be used to detect proviral DNA in circulating leukocytes. Due to the virus's variability, different PCR protocols provide variable sensitivity and some may not correctly detect all virus clades. Virus isolation is laborious and time-consuming, as it requires specialized expertise for co-cultivation of peripheral blood lymphocytes from suspected cats with primary feline T cells.[55]

Symptomatic cats should be administered supportive therapy to improve their general health. Administration of granulocyte (filgastrim), lymphocyte (insulin-like growth factor-I), and erythrocyte (erythropoietin) stimulating factors may be beneficial. Antiviral drugs, mostly developed against HIV, are available for specific treatment of FIV infection, although some antiretroviral molecules have a higher toxicity in cats than in humans. These include AZT (3′-azido-2′,3′-dideoxythymidine) at the dosage of 5 to 10 mg/kg twice daily and AMD3100 at the dosage of 0.5 mg/kg twice daily. Feline interferon-omega, which has been recently licensed in several countries, has no side effects and can be administered lifelong, but its efficacy is still debated. In contrast, human interferon-alpha has been shown to significantly improve the survival rates of FIV-infected cats.[55] A killed vaccine is available in some countries, but its efficacy is uncertain. The only practical measure to control FIV transmission is the strict separation of infected cats and neutering of FIV-positive males, especially in multicat households, breeding catteries, and shelters. Cats should be tested before being introduced in new environments and, subsequently, on a yearly basis, which should help isolation of infected animals.[55]

Feline Leukemia Virus

Feline leukemia virus (FeLV) is a *Gammaretrovirus* of domestic and nondomestic felids that is classified into 4 subtypes (A, B, C, and T) on the basis of the host cell spectrum. FeLV-A is acquired from the field; FeLV-B arises from recombination between FeLV-A and endogenous retroviral sequences (enFeLV); FeLV-C originates from a mutation in the *env* gene; and FeLV-T is characterized by T lymphotropism. Another virus, feline sarcoma virus (FeSV), is the result of recombination between subtype A and cancer-associated cellular genes.[63] FeLV is shed in high amounts in the saliva, the main source of infection, and is easily transmitted through close contact between infected and susceptible cats. Consequently, animals living in multicat households, shelters, and breeding catteries are highly exposed to FeLV infection due to sharing of food and water dishes, mutual grooming, and sharing of common litter areas. Vertical transmission occurs frequently through the transplacental route or licking during nursing. Latently infected queens may also transmit the virus to their offspring due to FeLV reactivation during pregnancy.[64] Mammary colonization, in the absence of FeLV antigenemia, may represent an efficient source of vertical transmission via milk.[65] Kittens from infected queens may test antigen negative for several weeks or months, becoming positive only when the virus commences to replicate.[64]

In horizontal infections, virus replicates in lymphoid tissues of the oropharynx after entry. In some cats with efficient immune responses (early regressors), the virus is rapidly cleared from infected tissues, preventing systemic spread. When the immune response is not optimal, a FeLV viremia develops within lymphocytes and monocytes. In some cases, cats test positive by antigen-detection methods but only after weeks or months of infection. More commonly, however, there is a transient viremia (antigenemia is more preferable), but cats never recover from FeLV infection, remaining latently infected due to the presence of FeLV provirus in circulating mononuclear cells. Such animals often remain clinically healthy lifelong, unless immunosuppression or chronic stress causes virus reactivation. In cats with minimal immune responses, the virus causes a persistent viremia (antigenemia), reaching the bone marrow and other target tissues and inducing FeLV-related clinical signs. Due to the slow disease progression, signs may appear even after several years of viremia.[63]

FeLV disease includes a variety of clinical forms that are directly or indirectly caused by the virus replication in lymphoid tissues and bone marrow. Immunosuppression is the main consequence of FeLV infection and leads to exacerbation of the clinical course of infections caused by mild pathogens such as *Mycoplasma hemofelis* and other feline hemoplasmas, *Crytpococcus* spp, *Toxoplasma gondii*, feline coronavirus, and calicivirus. In the late stages of infection, cats may develop different types of lymphomas and/or acute leukemias. A proportion of fibrosarcomas are associated with FeSV infection.[58,64]

Reproductive disorders can be observed in FeLV-infected queens. In utero infection can lead to fetal resorption, abortion, and neonatal death. Fetal resorption may be responsible for long periods of apparent infertility. Abortion occurs late in gestation with expulsion of normal-appearing fetuses and may be accompanied by bacterial endometritis. Kittens with perinatal infections may develop the "fading-kitten syndrome," which is characterized by an early fatal outcome due to failure to nurse, dehydration, hypothermia, and thymic atrophy.[64]

Due to the presence of "regressor cats," FeLV vaccination, and frequent production of antibodies against endogenous FeLV, serologic methods are not commonly used for FeLV diagnosis. Direct diagnosis is carried out by means of antigen- and nucleic acid–detection methods. ELISA and immunochromatographic tests detect a soluble protein (p27) in the blood or plasma that is produced in excess during active FeLV replication. Such tests are useful to diagnose the FeLV-associated clinical forms that are usually associated with virus replication in circulating mononuclear cells. However, the ELISA does not detect latent infections because of the lack of free p27 in the blood.[66,67] In addition, clinical forms induced by viral replication restricted to particular tissues (bone marrow, mammary glands, central nervous system) may be not diagnosed by antigen-detection methods. Gel-based and real-time PCR for proviral DNA detection are useful to identify cats with latent infection, although such animals may not develop FeLV-associated disease during their life. Reverse transcription (RT)-PCR and real-time RT-PCR detection of viral RNA produced by replicating virus in the saliva or other biological fluids may overcome these limitations, but, as antigen-detection methods, they cannot diagnose latent infections.[63]

Management of FeLV-diseased cats is difficult because of the variable clinical presentations. Supportive therapy consisting of fluid administration and blood transfusions should be considered in chronically infected animals. Corticosteroids should be avoided unless their administration is aimed to improve the food intake in the presence of chronic stomatitis. Antibiotics are required in the case of concurrent bacterial infections. As in the case of FIV, antiviral drugs may have severe side effects in cats. AZT and feline interferon-omega have been proved to improve the clinical and immunologic status, with increased quality of life and prolonged life expectancy in treated cats.[64,68,69]

Apart form the strict separation of infected cats, FeLV prophylaxis benefits from the availability of effective vaccines. Those vaccines have good efficacy in terms of protection from the clinical forms of disease, but none prevents FeLV infection.[70,71] In fact, several experiments have demonstrated that FeLV vaccination neither induces sterilizing immunity nor protects cats from infection.[71]

Felid Herpesvirus 1

Felid herpesvirus 1 (FeHV-1), a herpesvirus of the Alphaherpesvirinae subfamily, is responsible for a respiratory disease in domestic cats known as feline viral rhinotracheitis. The virus infects domestic cats and some wild felids and causes latent infections that are reactivated intermittently due to stress conditions, immunosuppression, or parturition, giving rise to viral shedding through oronasal and conjunctival secretions. Virus transmission occurs through direct contact with acutely infected cats and latently infected cats with virus reactivation, whereas indirect contact plays a role in shelters, breeding catteries, and multicat households. Newborn kittens usually become infected through contact with oronasal secretions of the queens. In utero infections have been reported only under experimental conditions.[72,73]

Unlike with CaHV-1, FeHV-1–induced abortion is rarely observed and seems to occur more from debilitating effects than to direct virus involvement.[74] Although a brief period of viremia occurs during FeHV-1 primary infection,[75] there are no reports of isolation from the aborted fetuses in the field cases. FeHV-1 infection in a specific pathogen free cat colony involved 51 pregnant queens, but only 1 animal had a partial abortion. However, 61% of kittens born to infected queens developed FeVH-1–induced respiratory disease.[76] Intravenous inoculation of queens in late gestation resulted in abortion, stillbirth, or generalized neonatal infections, whereas there was no effect on gestation after intranasal inoculation.[76,77] Analogously, virus isolation from the genital tract of the queens and the tissues of their aborted fetuses was obtained only after intravenous FeHV-1 inoculation. This unnatural route of infection was the only one causing necrotic lesions in the uterus, placenta, and vagina of the queens and in the liver of the fetuses. Congenital infection of kittens also has been achieved by FeHV-1 instillation in the vagina of pregnant queens. In this experiment, kittens died in the first 3 weeks of life as a consequence of generalized infection. They had fibrinosuppurative rhinotracheitis, bronchopneumonia, and multifocal hepatic necrosis at the time of necropsy, with viral inclusions in the respiratory epithelium and hepatocytes.[78]

FeHV-1 infection is commonly diagnosed by virus isolation, using oropharyngeal and conjunctival swab samples inoculated into feline cell lines, or by PCR-based methods. Conjunctival smears also may be examined by immunofluorescence. Treatment of feline viral rhinotracheitis is mainly supportive and may require antibiotic administration for concurrent bacterial infections.[72] Antiherpetic drugs (trifluridine, idoxuridine, ganciclovir, feline interferon-omega) are used only for the treatment of FeHV-1 ocular disease. FeHV-1 prophylaxis is based on vaccination using both MLV and inactivated formulations. Analogous to other herpesvirus vaccines, FeHV-1 vaccines protect against the clinical disease but not infection and shedding of virulent virus.[73]

SUMMARY

Several viruses have been associated with reproductive failures in dogs and cats. Parvoviruses (CMV and FPLV) and herpesviruses (CaHV and FeHV) can cause pregnancy losses and neonatal mortality in both domestic dogs and cats, often with different pathogenetic mechanisms according to the carnivore species. Sporadic BTV infection has been reported in pregnant bitches vaccinated with contaminated products that resulted in abortion and stillbirth. In cats, retroviral infections caused by FIV and FeLV are commonly responsible for in utero virus transmission and pregnancy losses. Effective treatment protocols consisting of administration of antiviral drugs and prophylactic measures based on vaccination of susceptible animals are available only for few viral diseases; whereas therapy and prevention of other viruses impacting on canine and feline pregnancy are currently lacking.

REFERENCES

1. Verstegen J, Dhaliwal G, Verstegen-Onclin K. Canine and feline pregnancy loss due to viral and non-infectious causes: a review. Theriogenology 2008;70:304–19.
2. Greene CE, Addie DD. Feline parvovirus infections. In: Greene CE, editor. Infectious diseases of the dog and cat. 3rd edition. St Louis: Saunders Elsevier; 2006. p. 78–88.
3. Decaro N, Martella V, Buonavoglia C. Canine adenoviruses and herpesvirus. Vet Clin North Am Small Anim Pract 2008;38:799–814.

4. Manteufel J, Truyen U. Animal bocaviruses: a brief review. Intervirology 2008;51: 328–34.
5. Minson AC, Davison A, Eberle R, et al. Family Herpesviridae. In: van Regenmortel MHV, Fauquet CM, Bishop DHL, et al, editors. Virus taxonomy. Seventh Report of the International Committee on Taxonomy of Viruses. New York: Academic Press; 2000. p. 203–25.
6. Carmichael LE. Herpesvirus canis: aspects of pathogenesis and immune response. J Am Vet Med Assoc 1970;156:1714–21.
7. Greene CE, Carmichael LE. Canine herpesvirus infection. In: Greene CE, editor. Infectious diseases of the dog and cat. 3rd edition. St Louis: Saunders Elsevier; 2006. p. 47–53.
8. Hashimoto A, Hirai K, Okada K, et al. Pathology of the placenta and newborn pups with suspected intrauterine infection of canine herpesvirus. Am J Vet Res 1979;40: 1236–40.
9. Buonavoglia C, Martella V. Canine respiratory viruses. Vet Res 2007;38:355–73.
10. Decaro N, Amorisco F, Desario C, et al. Development and validation of a real-time PCR assay for specific and sensitive detection of canid herpesvirus 1. J Virol Methods 2010;169:176–80.
11. Carmichael LE, Barnes FD, Percy DH. Temperature as a factor in resistance of young puppies to canine herpesvirus. J Infect Dis 1969;120:669–78.
12. Binn LN, Lazar EC, Eddy GA, et al. Recovery and characterization of a minute virus of canines. Infect Immun 1970;1:503–8.
13. Greene CE, Decaro N. Canine viral enteritis. In: Greene CE, editor. Infectious diseases of the dog and cat. 4th edition. Philadelphia: WB Saunders; 2012. p. 67–80.
14. Tattersall P, Bergoin M, Boom ME, et al. Family Parvoviridae. In: Fauquet CM, Mayo MA, Maniloff J, et al, editors. Virus taxonomy. Eighth Report of the International Committee on Taxonomy of Viruses. Amsterdam: Elsevier; 2005. p. 353–69.
15. Decaro N, Martella V, Desario C, et al. L'infezione del cane da parvovirus tipo 1 (CPV-1). Obiettivi e Documenti Veterinari 2008;XXIX:27–30.
16. Mochizuki M, Hashimoto M, Hajima T, et al. Virologic and serologic identification of minute virus of canines (canine parvovirus type 1) from dogs in Japan. J Clin Microbiol 2002;40:3993–8.
17. Carmichael LE. Canine parvovirus type 1 (minute virus of canines). In: Horzinek MC, series editor. Virus infections of vertebrates, Vol. I. Appel MJ, editor. Virus infections of varnivores. Amsterdam: Elsevier; 1987. p. 63–7.
18. Carmichael LE, Schlafer DH, Hashimoto A. Minute virus of canine (MCV, canine parvovirus type-1): pathogenicity for pups and seroprevalence estimate. J Vet Diagn Invest 1994;6:165–74.
19. Harrison LR, Styer EL, Pursell AR, et al. Fatal disease in nursing puppies associated with minute virus of canine. J Vet Diagn Invest 1992;4:19–22.
20. Jarpild B, Johansson H, Carmichael LE. A fatal case of pup infection with minute virus of canines (MVC). J Vet Diagn Invest 1996;8:484–7.
21. Pratelli A, Buonavoglia D, Tempesta M, et al. Fatal canine parvovirus type-1 infection in pups from Italy. J Vet Diagn Invest 1999;11:365–7.
22. Decaro N, Altamura M, Pratelli A, et al. Evaluation of the innate immune response in pups during canine parvovirus type 1 infection. New Microbiol 2002;25:291–8.
23. Eminaga S, Palus V, Cherubini GB. Minute virus as a possible cause of neurological problems in dogs. Vet Rec 2011;168:111–2.
24. Ohshima T, Kawakami K, Abe T, et al. A minute virus of canines (MVC: canine bocavirus) isolated from an elderly dog with severe gastroenteritis, and phylogenetic analysis of MVC strains. Vet Microbiol 2010;145:334–8.

25. Osburn BI. Bluetongue virus. Vet Clin North Am Food Anim Pract 1994;10:547–60.
26. Akita GY, Ianconescu M, MacLachlan NJ, et al. Bluetongue disease in dogs associated with contaminated vaccine. Vet Rec 1994;134:283–4.
27. Wilbur LA, Evermann JF, Levings RL, et al. Abortion and death in pregnant bitches associated with a canine vaccine contaminated with bluetongue virus. J Am Vet Med Assoc 1994;204:1762–5.
28. Brown CC, Rhyan JC, Grubman MJ, et al. Distribution of bluetongue virus in tissues of experimentally infected pregnant dogs as determined by in situ hybridization. Vet Pathol 1996;33:337–40.
29. Levings RL, Wilbur LA, Evermann JF, et al. Abortion and death in pregnant bitches associated with a canine vaccine contaminated with bluetongue virus. Dev Biol Stand 1996;88:219–20.
30. Alexander KA, MacLachlan NJ, Kat PW, et al. Evidence of natural bluetongue virus infection among African carnivores. Am J Trop Med Hyg 1994;51:568–76.
31. Decaro N, Buonavoglia C. Canine parvovirus: a review of epidemiological and diagnostic aspects, with emphasis on type 2c. Vet Microbiol 2012;155:1–12.
32. Decaro N, Desario C, Miccolupo A, et al. Genetic analysis of feline panleukopenia viruses from cats with gastroenteritis. J Gen Virol 2008;89:2290–8.
33. Shackelton LA, Parrish CR, Truyen U, et al. High rate of viral evolution associated with the emergence of carnivore parvovirus. Proc Natl Acad Sci USA 2005;102:379–84.
34. Decaro N, Desario C, Parisi A, et al. Genetic analysis of canine parvovirus type 2c. Virology 2009;385:5–10.
35. Buonavoglia C, Martella V, Pratelli A, et al. Evidence for evolution of canine parvovirus type-2 in Italy. J Gen Virol 2001;82:1555–60.
36. Truyen U, Evermann JF, Vieler E, et al. Evolution of canine parvovirus involved loss and gain of feline host range. Virology 1996;215:186–9.
37. Mochizuki M, Harasawa R, Nakatani H. Antigenic and genomic variabilities among recently prevalent parvoviruses of canine and feline origin in Japan. Vet Microbiol 1993;38:1–10.
38. Truyen U, Platzer G, Parrish CR. Antigenic type distribution among canine parvoviruses in dogs and cats in Germany. Vet Rec 1996;138:365–6.
39. Ikeda Y, Mochizuki M, Naito R, et al. Predominance of canine parvovirus (CPV) in unvaccinated cat populations and emergence of new antigenic types of CPVs in cats. Virology 2000;278:13–9.
40. Decaro N, Buonavoglia D, Desario C, et al. Characterisation of canine parvovirus strains isolated from cats with feline panleukopenia. Res Vet Sci 2010;89:275–8.
41. Decaro N, Desario C, Amorisco F, et al. Canine parvovirus type 2c infection in a kitten associated with intracranial abscess and convulsions. J Feline Med 2011;13:231–6.
42. Truyen U, Addie D, Belák S, et al. Feline panleukopenia. ABCD guidelines on prevention and management. J Feline Med Surg 2009;11:538–46.
43. Greene CE, Gorgasz EJ, Martin CL. Hydranencephaly associated with feline panleukopenia. J Am Vet Med Assoc 1982;180:767–8.
44. Sharp NJ, Davis BJ, Guy JS, et al. Hydranencephaly and cerebellar hypoplasia in two kittens attributed to intrauterine parvovirus infection. J Comp Pathol 1999;121:39–53.
45. Csiza CK, De Lahunta A, Scott FW, et al. Pathogenesis of feline panleukopenia virus in susceptible newborn kittens, II. Pathology and immunofluorescence. Infect Immun 1971;3:838–46.
46. Kilham L, Margolis G, Colby ED. Cerebellar ataxia and its congenital transmission in cats by feline panleukopenia virus. J Am Vet Med Assoc 1971;158(Suppl 2):888.

47. Decaro N, Elia G, Campolo M, et al. New approaches for the molecular characterization of canine parvovirus type 2 strains. J Vet Med B Infect Dis Vet Public Health 2005;52:316–9.
48. Decaro N, Elia G, Martella V, et al. Characterisation of the canine parvovirus type 2 variants using minor groove binder probe technology. J Virol Methods 2006;133: 92–9.
49. Decaro N, Elia G, Desario C, et al. A minor groove binder probe real-time PCR assay for discrimination between type 2-based vaccines and field strains of canine parvovirus. J Virol Methods 2006;136:65–70.
50. Decaro N, Martella V, Elia G, et al. Diagnostic tools based on minor groove binder probe technology for rapid identification of vaccinal and field strains of canine parvovirus type 2b. J Virol Methods 2006;138:10–6.
51. Decaro N, Desario C, Elia G, et al. Occurrence of severe gastroenteritis in pups after canine parvovirus vaccine administration: a clinical and laboratory diagnostic dilemma. Vaccine 2007;25:1161–6.
52. Decaro N, Desario C, Lucente MS, et al. Specific identification of feline panleukopenia virus and its rapid differentiation from canine parvoviruses using minor groove binder probes. J Virol Methods 2008;147:67–71.
53. Gamoh K, Senda M, Inoue Y, et al. Efficacy of an inactivated feline panleucopenia virus vaccine against a canine parvovirus isolated from a domestic cat. Vet Rec 2005;157: 285–7.
54. Dunham SP, Graham E. Retroviral infections of small animals. Vet Clin North Am Small Anim Pract 2008;38:879–901.
55. Hosie MJ, Addie D, Belák S, et al. Feline immunodeficiency. ABCD guidelines on prevention and management. J Feline Med Surg 2009;11:575–84.
56. Rogers AB, Hoover EA. Maternal-fetal feline immunodeficiency virus transmission: timing and tissue tropisms. J Infect Dis 1998;178:960–7.
57. Sellon RHartmann K. Feline immunodeficiency virus infection. In: Greene CE, editor. Infectious diseases of the dog and cat. 3rd edition. St Louis: WB Saunders; 2006. p. 131–42.
58. Hartmann K. Clinical aspects of feline immunodeficiency and feline leukemia virus infection. Vet Immunol Immunopathol 2011;143:190–1.
59. O'Neil LL, Burkhard MJ, Diehl LJ, et al. Vertical transmission of feline immunodeficiency virus. AIDS Res Hum Retroviruses 1995;11:171–82.
60. Rogers AB, Hoover EA. Fetal feline immunodeficiency virus is prevalent and occult. J Infect Dis 2002;186:895–904.
61. O'Neil LL, Burkhard MJ, Hoover EA. Frequent perinatal transmission of feline immunodeficiency virus by chronically infected cats. J Virol 1996;70:2894–901.
62. Weaver CC, Burgess SC, Nelson PD, et al. Placental immunopathology and pregnancy failure in the FIV-infected cat. Placenta 2005;26:138–47.
63. Lutz H, Addie D, Belák S, et al. Feline leukaemia. ABCD guidelines on prevention and management. J Feline Med Surg 2009;11:565–74.
64. Hartmann K. Feline leukemia virus infection. In: Greene CE, editor. Infectious diseases of the dog and cat. 3rd edition. St Louis: WB Saunders; 2006. p. 105–31.
65. Pacitti AM, Jarrett O, Hay D. Transmission of feline leukaemia virus in the milk of a non-viraemic cat. Vet Rec 1986;118:381–4.
66. Lutz H, Pedersen N, Higgins J, et al. Humoral immune reactivity to feline leukemia virus and associated antigens in cats naturally infected with feline leukemia virus. Cancer Res 1980;40:3642–51.

67. Hartmann K, Griessmayr P, Schulz B, et al. Quality of different in-clinic test systems for feline immunodeficiency virus and feline leukaemia virus infection. J Feline Med Surg 2007;9:439–45.
68. Hartmann K, Donath A, Beer B, et al. Use of two virustatica (AZT, PMEA) in the treatment of FIV and of FeLV seropositive cats with clinical symptoms. Vet Immunol Immunopathol 1992;35:167–75.
69. de Mari K, Maynard L, Sanquer A, et al. Therapeutic effects of recombinant feline interferon-omega on feline leukemia virus (FeLV)-infected and FeLV/feline immunodeficiency virus (FIV)-coinfected symptomatic cats. J Vet Intern Med 2004;18: 477–82.
70. Kensil CR, Barrett C, Kushner N, et al. Development of a genetically engineered vaccine against feline leukemia virus infection. J Am Vet Med Assoc 1991;199: 1423–7.
71. Hofmann-Lehmann R, Cattori V, Tandon R, et al. Vaccination against the feline leukaemia virus: outcome and response categories and long-term follow-up. Vaccine 2007;25:5531–9.
72. Gaskell R, Dawson S, Radford A, et al. Feline herpesvirus. Vet Res 2007;38:337–54.
73. Thiry E, Addie D, Belák S, et al. Feline herpesvirus infection. ABCD guidelines on prevention and management. J Feline Med Surg 2009;11:547–55.
74. Gaskell RM, Dawson S. Viral-induced upper respiratory tract disease. In: Chandler EA, Gaskell CJ, Gaskell RM, editors. Feline medicine and therapeutics. Oxford (UK): Blackwell Scientific Publications; 1994. p. 453–72.
75. Westermeyer HD, Thomasy SM, Kado-Fong H, et al. Assessment of viremia associated with experimental primary feline herpesvirus infection or presumed herpetic recrudescence in cats. Am J Vet Res 2009;70:99–104.
76. Hoover EA, Griesemer RA. Experimental feline herpesvirus infection in the pregnant cat. Am J Pathol 1971;65:173–88.
77. Johnson RT. The pathogenesis of herpes virus encephalitis. II. A cellular basis for the development of resistance with age. J Exp Med 1964;120:359–74.
78. Bittle JL, Peckham JC. Genital infection induced by feline rhinotracheitis virus and effects on newborn kittens. J Am Vet Med Assoc 1971;158(Suppl 2):927–8.

Index

Note: Page numbers of article titles are in **boldface** type.

Vet Clin Small Anim 42 (2012) 599–614
doi:10.1016/S0195-5616(12)00044-7
vetsmall.theclinics.com
0195-5616/12/$ – see front matter

M

U

V

ELSEVIER